ON BEHALF OF CHILDREN

ON BEHALF
OF CHILDREN

William Hetznecker, M.D.

Associate Professor of Psychiatry,
Temple University Health Sciences Center;
Staff Psychiatrist,
St. Christopher's Hospital for Children;
formerly Director, Children and Family Unit,
Temple University Community Mental Health Center,
Philadelphia, Penna.

Marc A. Forman, M.D.

Associate Professor of Psychiatry and Pediatrics,
Temple University Health Sciences Center;
Director, Child Psychiatry Center
at St. Christopher's Hospital for Children,
Philadelphia, Penna.

With a Foreword by

Leon Eisenberg, M.D.

GRUNE & STRATTON
A Subsidiary of Harcourt Brace Jovanovich, Publishers
New York   San Francisco   London

Library of Congress Cataloging in Publication Data
Hetznecker, William.
    On Behalf of Children.
    Includes bibliographical references.
    1. Child mental health. I. Forman, Marc A.,
joint author. II. Title. [DNLM: 1. Child psychi-
atry. 2. Community mental health services. WS350
H59lo 1974]
RJ111.H47   362.2   74-8454
ISBN 0-8089-0844-8

Grune & Stratton, Inc.
111 Fifth Avenue
New York, New York 10003

Library of Congress Catalog Card Number 74-8454
International Standard Book Number 0-8089-0844-8
Printed in the United States of America

To Noreen and Phyllis
With Love

Contents

PART III   New Manpower Resources

PART IV   Overview

Foreword

This is a most unusual book, refreshing in its candor, distinguished by its compassion, and stimulating in its penetrating analysis of the daily problems of professional work on a community level. It is rare, indeed, for two clinicians, who retain their enthusiasm for their work with children, to begin their account by describing two "failed" cases rather than by presenting the successes that they could as readily have selected from their case files. But they, and we, learn from those "failures." The new methods they introduce in their metamorphosis to community work might very well have made the difference in outcome for the "traditional" pattern of treatment of the middle class family in the first case excerpt. Yet these additional inputs proved insufficient as remedies for the multiproblem family whose members require still more in the way of social supports and innovation. Quite eloquently, the authors have warned us at the outset that they have no nostrums to sell, no cure-alls to offer, no oversimplifications to provide. Here and there they report modest gains and elsewhere note what must have been dispiriting losses; yet they continue to strive, with courage and concern, on behalf of children and families who face overwhelming obstacles. Note well that they *continue to strive*—for the bane of programs for the poor has been the frequency with which they have been abandoned by professionals who can choose, as the poor cannot, an easier path to status and prestige.

What distinguishes this book is the authors' ability to reflect on their own experience and to turn adversity to advantage by dissecting out the factors, often extraneous to the clinical program itself, that made for either the viability or curtailment of apparently well-thought-out activities. Although they have undertaken a systematic evaluation of their

most durable innovation (the Incentive Specialist Program), that evaluation is not yet complete and hence not reported here. They are right,
however, to focus on how out-reach programs may be gotten underway
and what it takes to keep them going, even before it is possible to find out
if they benefit the target population. For, the best idea is no idea if it cannot get off the ground and be kept going long enough to provide the basis
for an estimate of its effectiveness. Evaluation of outcome is rare enough
in community mental health; fresh ideas are even rarer; and innovators
are all too often stymied by institutional barriers to change. Bill
Hetznecker and Marc Forman offer us, not a how-to-do-it, but a what-
to-watch-out-for, in trying to construct services for the urban poor.

They are clearly committed to efforts to diminish the suffering of
those victimized by society. The contemporary radical thrust in mental
health questions the very propriety of such undertakings, arguing that
the goal is to eliminate the social conditions that produce the victims, not
to put bandaids on their wounds. Before we are persuaded, the metaphor
demands closer inspection. If we are merely putting bandaids on deep
wounds, then the analysis is appropriate. But if we are cleaning and su-
turing wounds that would otherwise become infected and be left gaping,
then we are obligated to intervene. This does not relieve us of the
responsibility to try to blunt or remove the knives that produce the
wounds. But the casualties are *people* and *their* wounds will not disappear, even if we are successful in diminishing the attack on others.

Let us consider similar examples. Certain vaccines can almost
totally eliminate the risk of acquiring particular diseases. Inequities in
the distribution of medical care (as well as failures in the education of
parents on the necessity for such care) have led to a situation in which
minority children have vaccination rates far lower than those for the
population at large. Would anyone seriously argue that it is wrong to
provide curative services to the unvaccinated who do fall ill because that
would undercut the campaign for universal vaccination? Consider a
second case. Complications of pregnancy and parturition—complications which occur at far greater rates among mothers who are of low
socioeconomic status, under age, and from minority groups—result in
increased risk of brain damage among their offspring. Should we not
provide remedial and corrective service for such handicapped children
even as we speak out for proper preventive measures that might have ob-
viated those brain insults? The mental health team that evaluates and
plans therapeutic programs for mentally defective and brain damaged
children endeavors to minimize the impact on youngsters for whom
primary prevention is no longer a meaningful issue.

It has long been recognized as a public health principle that the
identification of a child with tuberculosis must spur a search for family
contacts at the very same time that treatment is initiated for the index
case. Similarly, the discovery of lead poisoning mandates a thorough

study of family housing. The latter example is peculiarly instructive. A vigorous national housing program would do much to prevent lead poisoning (not all, since environmental sources of lead other than paint exist). The physician who sees the ravages of lead poisoning has a responsibility as a citizen to take the lead in pressing the case for better housing. However, there is much he can do to diminish the impact on actual and potential victims through screening programs for early identification and measures for prompt treatment. No one who is at all realistic about the nature and severity of our current housing problem anticipates that slum housing will be replaced within any short-run time frame; thus, social responsibility involves taking action for secondary prevention in the midst of the fight for primary prevention.

But the radical critique is not quite so readily dismissed. "Services" can be a sop to public conscience when they are too little and too late. Hanging out a public sign and announcing a "service" substitutes symbol for reality; it may indeed defuse public urgency for appropriately directed action. In mental health, we are called upon to consult, as the authors were, to welfare agencies in helping to manage the problems of foster children. What we often find are disturbed children for whom traditional remedies might be expected to be helpful *if* the living situation of the children were stabilized and *if* the remedies were made available. All too often, neither condition obtains. The inadequate rates of subsidy for foster parents, the excessively large case loads of welfare workers, and the fiction that the child is not adoptable because he has living parents (even though they have abandoned him in all but name) keep him in limbo, at home nowhere. The recommended psychological treatment is either not to be had from mental health clinics, or time and transportation problems preclude his getting to the clinic, day treatment, or recreation program. For a consultant to permit the fiction that there is a "psychiatric service" for foster children under such circumstances verges on the fraudulent. Such "service" is all too often packaged and sold as a cheap way out of the real need for the development of functional services to (1) maintain families when they are salvageable; (2) provide stable and loving foster care when there is hope of reestablishing family bonds temporarily severed; and (3) initiate action to ensure adoption when family bonds cannot be restored. A consultant who dictates his note for the chart, collects his fee, and makes no effort to evaluate the impact of his role helps "cool the mark out."

The authors, well aware of the Scylla and Charybdis of mental health work, share with us their experience in trying to steer their vessel between the hazards of an exclusive focus on "treatment" or "prevention." The day-to-day choices are difficult ones. If one insists from the start on optimal conditions for an effective program, one may never get a program started; if one is trapped into too much compromise, the program may be doomed before it begins. The easiest position to adopt is one of moral superiority by refusing to make the compromises demanded by the politics of the public sector, but that position must be recognized for what it is: an abandonment of society's victims. The authors refuse to allow themselves the luxury of remaining above the fray.

None of this is new, either to medicine or psychiatry. The physician is called upon to treat illness, a phenomenon with social no less than biological roots. This paradox is clearly evident in the contributions of the great pathologist, Rudolf Virchow. Virchow is celebrated in medical history as the founder of the doctrine of cellular pathology. This doctrine, along with the germ theory of disease, provided the foundation in the latter half of the 19th century for what we proudly hail as "scientific medicine." In its current version, scientific medicine has become so preoccupied with cell and organ dysfunction in the individual that it may be blind to the social factors that have generated those dysfunctions. It has been forgotten that our hero, Virchow, was a champion of social medicine as well.

In the summer of 1847, Upper Silesia was the scene of an epidemic of relapsing fever. The central government in Berlin was forced to form a Commission of Investigation, with Virchow as one of its members. He immediately recognized the social sources of the epidemic and his recommendation for public health measures emphasized the necessity for "complete and unrestricted democracy." His report concluded: "All the world knows that the proletariat of our day has been mainly brought into existence by the introduction and improvement of machinery; that in proportion as agriculture, manufacture, navigation and land transport have acquired an unprecedented extension, manpower has completely lost its autonomy; human beings have become incorporated as mere cogwheels in machine enterprise—living cogwheels indeed, but treated as of no more value than dead matter. The human instruments are regarded as mere 'hands'! Are the triumphs of human genius to lead only to this: that the human race should become more miserable? Unquestionably not. The object of our century must be to reduce to the utmost the purely mechanical parts of human activity. Man should work only as much as needful to wrest from the soil whatever is indispensible to provide a comfortable life for the whole race; but he should not waste his best energies in producing capital. Capital is a title to enjoyment; but why should this title be increased to a degree beyond all reason? . . . At the least, capital and labor power must have equal rights, and living energies must no longer be subordinate to dead capital."

Virchow's report was issued in 1848, a year of social revolution in Europe. Indeed, he founded a journal with the title "Medical Reform." When reaction set in, he lost his salary and his office at the Charité. It was not until 1856 that the growing fame of his work led to his recall to Berlin. Though he remained in the political left, his energies and efforts centered more on the formulation of a scientific basis for the understanding of disease. Coopted? Perhaps, but we must also recognize that his scientific work provided society with the fundamental groundwork for our enormous technical capacities in overcoming disease.

Psychiatry itself has swung between emphases on the social and the biological. Nothing illustrates this more clearly than the factors behind the present great improvement in our ability to manage acute psychosis. On the one hand, these stem directly from the movement for "moral treatment of the insane" which began at the time of the French Revolution and, on the other, from the development in the last 25 years of powerful psychotropic drugs. But good hospital care and the appropriate use of medication suffice only to reverse the dramatic manifestations of psychotic distress; the patient requires psychological support, continuing medical care, opportunities for meaningful work, decent housing, and reintegration into the community if his or her life is to have any chance of being a satisfying one. Neither our patients nor the mental health professions can afford the either/or of *the* social or *the* medical model of illness. It is as absurd to deny the mounting evidence of a genetic diathesis for schizophrenia and manic-depressive disease as it is to ignore the role of social forces in the precipitation of individual episodes and in their resolution. It is an intolerable diversion of our common energies from the task at hand to trumpet causal exclusionism when the real challenge is the development of an effective response to each patient's needs, a response which makes opportunistic use of every measure that can be devised.

It is precisely this search for a way through the maze of social and environmental conflicts and contradictions that infuses the work I am privileged to introduce. The authors share their travails with their co-workers, their community, and with us. They disdain no avenue that promises relief for the distress of others. Nor do they blink at the barriers that bestride the road. They tell it as it is. They are under no illusions that they have made more than a beginning. But they *have* made that beginning. And they continue to build on it, in the very midst of this era of malign neglect.

I owe the reader a final paragraph in the spirit of a reasonable requirement for full disclosure. I know the authors. I do have warm feelings for them both. I met Marc in the course of a visit to St. Christopher's and at once recognized his clinical acumen, his commitment, and his capacity for insightful analysis. Bill is a man whose religious convictions guide his life as powerfully out of church as in. In his sensitivity, his concern, and his intellectual mastery, he embodies the best attributes of the physician. He was a resident of mine when I headed the Children's Psychiatric Service at the Johns Hopkins Hospital. I can make no acknowledgment with greater pride.

Leon Eisenberg, M.D.
Professor of Psychiatry, Harvard Medical School

So here I am, in the middle way, having had twenty years—
Twenty years largely wasted, the years of l'entre deux guerres—
Trying to learn to use words, and every attempt
Is a wholly new start, and a different kind of failure
Because one has only learnt to get the better of words
For the thing one no longer has to say, or the way in which
One is no longer disposed to say it. And so each venture
Is a new beginning, a raid on the inarticulate
With shabby equipment always deteriorating
In the general mess of imprecision of feeling,
Undisciplined squads of emotion.

T. S. ELIOT

Preface

This book is not the last nor the final, but simply one version of the latest word. Our view is tentative and partial—qualities determined by the character of experience itself. What and how we think is founded initially on the process of becoming physicians. Subsequently, we developed the knowledge and skills of clinical psychiatrists. We were strongly influenced by psychoanalytic theory and dynamically oriented therapy. Our medical and psychiatric training had emphasized the individual, and specifically the internal workings of the individual.

The importance of social events and concepts which formed the mainstay of our thinking entered our lives in different ways. For one, (Dr. Forman) service as a psychiatrist in the Air Force revealed how a relatively closed society strongly affected not only how individuals adapted, but determined what was maladaptation and what a psychiatrist could and could not do. For the other, (Dr. Hetznecker) service in Indian Health and later exposure to epidemiologic thinking demonstrated vividly the influence of class and culture on the occurrence of illness and the capacity to determine one's destiny. For both, child psychiatric training meant day-to-day involvement with parents, teachers, and counselors—the social world of the child.

Through our individual sojourns, we arrived at the strongly held conviction that teaching of medicine must broaden and expand widely outward as effectively as it narrows and delves deeply inward. Social science instruction, but more important, the social perspective on human life, health, and illness should be essential at every step in medical education. We hold that an integrated curriculum including the sweep of social science from history and anthropology to social psychology and public administration are more important in the formation of the mind of a physician than cell biology or gross anatomy.

W. H.
M. A. F.

Acknowledgments

Authors often write that they are indebted to so many people that they cannot acknowledge all of them. Contrary to the usual practice, we wish to cite the contributions of many who were important in our development and in the making of this book. We gratefully acknowledge those whose lives we share and who sustained us with their belief, in the hope that they will be pleased by this book: our wives, our parents, Mary, and our children Alyssa, Billy, Bob, Dan, James, Matt, Paul, Sarah, and Victoria; our teachers, who taught us more than we could learn: John M. Dunn, Leon Eisenberg, Roger D. Freeman, Elmer A. Gardner, Ariel Loewy, B. Perry Ottenberg, Myrtle L. Pleune, Dane G. Prugh, Alijandro Rodriguez, John Romano, Calvin F. Settlage.

We thank our colleagues and friends with whom we worked and on whom we depended: Millie Thompson Bailey, Phil Band, Betsy Berger, Dave Berger, Ted Blunt, Don Bruce, Corrina Caldwell, Marge Eckert, Fred Glaser, Anne Glass, Jan Porter Gump, Skip Gump, Dick Hanusey, Lou Harris, Christine Kennedy, Nancy Lonsinger, Paul McIlhenny, Norm Newberg, Tony Panzetta, Matilde Salganicoff, Barbara Scott, Althris Shirdan, Florence Silverblatt, Gerard Weber and Paul Wender, as well as the Black Brothers, Incentive Specialists, Mental Health Assistants, the staff of Children and Family Division of the Philadelphia Department of Public Welfare, and the staffs of the Children and Family Unit and the Child Psychiatry Center.

We are grateful to our patrons, Paul Kotin, R. Bruce Sloane, Victor C. Vaughan, III, whose permission for our study leave made this book possible; to the staff of the Haverford College Library, who provided office space and kind hospitality; to Joan Sharp, our secretary and typist, who transformed our boring tapes and rambling drafts into an elegant manuscript; and to our editors at Grune & Stratton who guided us through the maze of bookmaking, Doreen Berne and Caryl Snapperman.

We wish to acknowledge the kind cooperation of John H. Diamond, Principal, Hartranft Elementary School, and Beatrice M. Taliaferro in permitting us to publish the cover photograph which was taken by Marc A. Forman.

For their authorship of Chapters 6 and 9, which add important dimensions to this book, we specifically acknowledge Bari Blumenstein, L. Wayne Higley, Robert J. Stewart, and Glenn Taylor. At the time of this work, Mr. Higley was Director, School Consultation and Mental Retardation Services, Temple Community Mental Health Center, and Mrs. Blumenstein was Psychoeducational Specialist at the Temple Community Mental Health Center, Philadelphia, Penna. Mr. Higley is currently Director, Partial Hospitalization Services, Philadelphia Child Guidance Clinic; Mrs. Blumenstein is presently Psychoeducational Specialist, Child Psychiatry Center at St. Christopher's Hospital for Children, Philadelphia, Penna. Dr. Stewart is Assistant Clinical Director, Child Psychiatry Center, and Mr. Taylor is Director of the Black Brother Program at the Child Psychiatry Center.

We are grateful to the Philadelphia Foundation for its generous support of the consultation program to the Department of Public Welfare. The research aspects of the Incentive Specialist Program were supported in part by a grant from the U.S. Department of Health, Education, and Welfare, Mental Health Services Development Branch (5R01-MH-18134).

Names of children, families, and schools cited in case examples in this book are fictitious, but refer to actual persons, places, and events.

1

Perspective

A STATEMENT OF THE PROBLEM

Our culture is in conflict about its children. We sentimentalize about childhood, but we do little for children, especially for those children who need help. At all levels, health, educational, and welfare programs for children are inadequately funded, and yet we piously speak of children as our "future" and our "legacy." Our bequest to them, however, is symbolized by the welfare shelter, the dole, the detention center, and the state institution. Even though children represent our largest minority group, they have little political influence. Children do not vote, and lobbying efforts on their behalf frequently eventuate in too little, too late. Contrary to the popular aphorism, children are neither seen nor heard.

Within the mental health field, the report of the Joint Commission on Mental Health of Children documents in considerable detail the magnitude of the problem facing us.[1] There are millions of children who are already showing signs of emotional distress and more at-risk for the development of severe difficulties in the future. The report clearly delineates the dimensions of the problem and pointedly describes the woeful lack of available resources and remedies. The lengthy list of recommendations in the report, comprising the first 136 pages, represents an indictment of a culture which, despite its protestations, appears to ignore the needs of children. In turn, the Group for the Advancement of Psychiatry criticized the report because it made "no attempt to understand the underlying factors in our confusing attitudes toward children."[2]

What are these underlying factors? At both the cultural and personal levels, they appear to be an admixture of conflicting belief systems and realities. Our culture gives high status to values such as freedom, individual initiative, independence, mobility, economic progress, and success. Yet, the presence of children and the caretaking tasks which they require serve as impediments to the adults' quest of desired goals. Our culture supports an individualistic ethic, but we frequently deal with children in small groups, for example, the family, the gang, the classroom. We value democracy as well as authority, and we must somehow try to balance these competing notions within our family structure. Our culture promotes youthfulness in fashion and manners, but as adults get older, children are a reminder of their lost youth. Privacy, quiet, and neatness are treasured by grownups, but children are noisy, messy intruders. And in a society dominated by the work ethic, children "have it easy," and are not in any sense an economic asset.

At the more personal level, we hold some long-standing myths and deep-seated feelings about children. Children are viewed either as dangerous, irrational animals, or they are romanticized into innocent little flowers and toys. They serve as caricatures of our own faults and traits, and often act out our infantile desires and needs. They compete for the love and attention of our spouses, and are sometimes victorious. They are seen as a "mistake" or a possession—although the question of who they really belong to is highlighted in situations of child abuse, abortion, and custody.

On the whole, then, children have one overriding fault when measured against our prevailing values—they "get in the way." As obstructions, children as a group share the same psychological space as the sick, the handicapped, the indigent, the mentally ill, prisoners, and the aged. If a child is also sick, chronically ill, mentally disturbed, behaviorally deviant, he is even more in the way. He is in double jeopardy. When someone is in the way, he is a hindrance, a bother, but we can do several things: Go around him; go over him; get him out of the way; or act as if he were not there. And that, all too frequently, is what we do to children. Of course, we also love, pamper, support, nourish, and spoil our children. But it is the negative side of our ambivalence which must be acknowledged and remedied if we are to fulfill our commitment to all of our children.

THE AIMS OF THIS BOOK

This book is about our work with children over the past 8 years. It is also about our work in clinics, schools, and agencies that take care of children. All of the book concerns programs that we developed, programs which we thought would be beneficial to children and their families. In describing these programs, we have tried to be specific, practical, and honest. We are sharing our successes and failures, false starts and small triumphs. Throughout our work, we have consistently asked the question: "What can we do that is realistic and sensible on behalf of the mental health needs of children?" Or perhaps, in a less grandiose fashion, the question should read, "What can two child psychiatrists, working with a limited budget and staff complement, do to help some children more than they have been helped before?"

In this book we will not review in any comprehensive fashion the entire field of child mental health. We will not discuss therapy, at least in the traditional way that term has been used. We will, however, describe action: the interventions we made and the programs we developed.

OUR POINT OF VIEW

All practice derives from prior conceptions, speculations, hunches, and biases—all of which constitute a "theory." Our own conceptual framework is basically a social-adaptational one, growing out of our experience in dynamic psychiatry, and influenced by ideas borrowed from sociology, transactional analysis, learning theory, and public health. Our viewpoint is not of the status of a "model," but it represents one way of looking at phenomena.

One can consider a spectrum of alternative ways of viewing disturbed behavior. We list these views in order from the more strict biological definition of mental illness at one end of the scale to essentially a nonillness definition at the other. All these alternatives are concerned with disturbed behavior in a person as he manifests it.

1. Mental illness is a "true" illness. The causes are internal, physiological, and molecular. The processes of the illness affect structure and function, though not necessarily in a measurable way, given the present diagnostic tools in use. The underlying internal causes significantly influence the person's behavior through primarily neurobiological means. An example of such an illness is neurosyphilis.
2. Mental illness is considered an illness which is formed, or arises, as a result of an interaction between the constitutional, hereditary endowment of the person and the human and nonhuman environment in which he functions. It is contingent on both of these major factors. Certain of the schizophrenias are examples.[3,4] This is the most commonly held disease model in modern medicine today.
3. Mental illness is distress which is primarily internal and subjective.

The person is a victim of psychologically determined conflict. Much of the battlefield in which this conflict rages is beyond the patient's awareness or control. The patient has a primary difficulty in his psychological response to perceptions; he is a victim of poor perception. Examples are the classical neuroses, the autoplastic conditions. In this view, definitive evidence of abnormal genetics, anatomy, or physiology has not been consistently or reliably demonstrated. This is the predominant outlook of the various psychodynamically based theories.

4. Mental illness is primarily and essentially behavior and is learned. This is basically a nonillness or nonmedical view of mental disturbance. The subject in this case is not a victim, but a student. Others, however, may be victims of his behavior. Social transmission, rather than biological factors are important.[5]

5. Finally, a social view that seems to be used more by social critics, professional writers, and those in the counterculture movement formulates that all society is sick. All individual illness is therefore an epiphenomenon. Once again, the person is a victim and, in fact, all persons in one way or another are victims of this ubiquitous social sickness that somehow affects society like smog.

One of the major risks in the overall medical or health-illness conceptualizations is that all behavior comes to be viewed in health-illness terms, leading to a view of the person as not responsible for his life and behavior to greater or lesser degrees. The word "illness" itself conveys the sense of being in the grip of something, of being passive. This is reflected in the statement that the person "just can't help himself." Frequently, a coexisting notion maintains that mental disturbance is due to a fault or sin. These are ambivalently held beliefs which represent a two-edged sword when applied to mental illness. Hazards such as these can occur especially under the first three options. There is, nevertheless, enough in the theory, practice, and experience of mental health workers of all kinds to justify the choice of any one of these views both on the basis of what one believes as well as what one does or has experienced. Any one view may apply, may be applied differently, and all have somewhat different therapeutic implications. The more strictly medical view has prevailed for recent historical, cultural, and certainly economic reasons.[6,7]

Our approach has been to settle on a modified social transactional model that is closely related to option 4 above. However, we subscribe to a more complicated model that includes intrapersonal, affective, and cognitive features.

We can consider any problem of human behavior from several levels of organization. These include the molecular, the systemic, the molar or organismic, and the social or interpersonal. The way in which one looks at a problem is determined in part by the level of organization examined. This level of organization, in turn, reciprocally determines the sorts of tools or instruments, terms and concepts one uses to examine that level. There needs to be a relative appropriateness between the method of viewing, the object being viewed, and the concepts or notions used to explain, organize, and interpret what is viewed.

An example may make this clear. A hand lens is used to enlarge those objects which are essentially visible to the naked eye, but it is of little use to examine in detail an individual cell. Neither is a microscope of great value in looking at the gross anatomy of a cockroach. In pursuing this matter, we can call to mind the simultaneous restriction of the extent of view as well as the enhancement of the details of view whenever we add an artificial lens system such as a microscope or telescope to aid our natural vision. Restriction and enhancement occur simultaneously with different aspects of the viewpoint.

Having chosen the social level of organization as the most useful conceptual space for viewing community mental health and related fields, we find ourselves among those who construe human activities in interpersonal, interactional, and transactional terms.[8-10] This view, if not the specific terminology in all cases, has been applied to the basic dyad of mother-infant behavior, and to the family.[11-14] The foundation for these relationships are conditioned by bonds of blood, affection, and law.

The same concept can be applied to the neighborhood and the peer group, which are more fortuitous and arbitrary associations. These relationships are governed by features of common living space, face-to-face familiarity, and cooperative activities that share ends and means.[15] Examples are the play activities of children, and formal and informal neighborhood groups.

Finally, we can apply such a view to larger, artificial social groupings which manifest varying degrees of permanence and interpersonal closeness. Such groups include church, school, places of work, and hospitals. Persons belonging to these groups may share some or all of the following: common beliefs, needs, goals, skills or deficits, and common personal characteristics such as gender and age.[16,17]

This social level of organization is precisely the arena of public health. The public health viewpoint includes interest and responsibility for both the well and the sick. In the notion of catchment area, derived from public health, there is a fixing of responsibility on the public health agency for the care of a geographically defined population. This notion also implies outreach and changes the nature of the health contract from an illness one with a primary responsibility on the consumer to a health-illness orientation with the prime responsibility on the dispenser of care. Another public health term is that of *population at-risk*. This signifies a defined group of people who have some probability of contracting an illness or disease because of certain characteristics inherent in the population or in certain conditions under which they live. Such a population because of a concomitance of various factors, constitutional and environmental, or both, have a higher than expected probability of contracting a disease or disturbance. For example, poor women who do not have adequate prenatal care are more likely to have infants at-risk for incurring maladies included under the term "spectrum of reproductive casualties."[18] Certainly, the concept of prevention has been taken over from public health by mental health. We will explore its implications and limitations in Chapter 12.

At this point, a brief aside is in order to make clear some underlying concepts without any attempt at detailed elaboration or theory building. In general, we see the notion of transaction as Spiegel derives it from Dewey and Bentley as a general term relating to the "mutually regulated processes of a system."[19] These processes are "reciprocal and reverberating." In casting our view primarily in the social field, we view interpersonal relationships as crucial. These vary in degree of intimacy, influence, and importance. For us, interaction connotes the emphasis on two or more parties who are involved with each other. The focus is on the *persons*, whereas the word transaction emphasizes the *process* of what is going on between them.

Basic to our view is the idea of *exchange*. In the process of a transaction, something is exchanged. It can be material or symbolic, verbal or gestural, explicit or implicit. Such an exchange can take place at any level of organization or it can involve several levels. The exchange can be purely internal (within the person), interpersonal, or sociocultural. A goal of an exchange is some type of balance of trade-offs.[20] Life may be viewed as a series of myriad deals and bargains, some with ourselves, some with others, some clear and explicit, some vague and implicit.

The notion of *contract* which we use throughout this book arises from this transactional exchange fundament. A contract is more verbalized and formal than an exchange, and it serves as the basis of negotiations between persons and groups. Such negotiations can be around everything from basic issues of affection, nurturance, and sexual exchange to more complex and specialized social contracts such as those involved in psychotherapy, consultation, and education. The notion of contract is part of a social adaptational focus which states that what goes on between the skins of individuals is more important than what goes on inside the skins of individuals. Clearly, at the operational level, neat phrases and contrasts do not apply. What goes on inside an individual person or group of persons is obviously reflected outside in what goes on between them. We have chosen to emphasize the latter.

In using the social adaptational view throughout this book, we recurrently invoke several additional concepts: social role and rule. *Social role* particularly includes those aspects of behavior which relate to expectations, performances, values, and concerns regarding status, power, and approval. Problems may be expressed as manifestations of role conflict, role confusion, role diffusion, and role competition. The concept of *rule* supplements that of role. Rule is seen as an organizing construct for the individual person or group. Rules are used to determine a particular role behavior in a given situation. Rules indicate what is and what is not approved performance and contain sanctions that are used to encourage conformity and discourage nonconformity. There are implicit as well as explicit rules for all social organizations: two-party transactions, family, peer group, school, or larger groups. It is important to emphasize that the use of these concepts is not to be taken as an evaluative a priori. We are not contending that the rules and roles of a particular social organization are the best or most appropriate way for people to behave and perform. These concepts, issues, and data are just one way of organizing the field for the mental health worker.

The above is a profile of how we use terms and what we will emphasize. We are not in any way contending that our viewpoint, concepts, and definitions are the truest and best (although for us, we clearly think that they are at present because we choose to use them). We do contend that we find them useful in both understanding what goes on and in guilding us in what to do about it. Since we cannot control how we are heard but only what we say, we want to disclaim, if possible, erroneous inference. By choosing the social level of organization and such social concepts as described above, there is, for the careless minded, the implication that other levels of organization or concepts related to them, for example, individual-intrapsychic, are wrong, bad, or out of date. This is a gratuitous inference. From the point of view of theorists, we are allowed the same free and arbitrary choice as the artist to decide which viewpoint we will use to guide our thinking and actions. The explicit meaning of choosing one viewpoint as opposed to another concerns the issues of usefulness and coherence, and not those of good and bad, or even necessarily those of true and false. The choice of one set of concepts over another may run the risk of incompleteness or preciousness. Given these possibilities, truth or falsity may be imputed, but the more strict judgement of truth or falsity is related to the internal consistency of the concepts within the framework that has been chosen and the empirical predictability of hypotheses that may derive from the framework.

For the most part, theorizing in psychological and behavioral areas is not such that any one theory can claim preeminence in its predictive value across a whole range of human behavior. We need to be satisfied with partial theories that relate to certain segments of human development, adaptation, and behavior. To formulate everything under the canopy of a unitary theory, explaining all or predicting outcomes at all levels of organization, is to be a knave or a fool, a dreamer or a zealot. In many instances, theoretical formulations in behavioral sciences are communication vehicles that we use to talk to each other in a somewhat coded manner. There is a fundamental distinction between the way we think or talk about something and what is *really* going on. Theories in the behavioral sciences do have some usefulness in terms of organizing and communicating knowledge. Their power of explanation and prediction is much weaker.

DEFINITIONS

The use of language brings with it competitive naming and labeling functions. Perhaps Adam and Eve's first arguments were over the "real" and "right" names for the animals. Such disputes neglect the various denotative, connotative, logical, and real differences between terms and things. In addition, one man's denotation is another's connotation. One man's substantial distinction is for another an accidental or lesser characteristic. We are all involved at times in a babel. We use terms interchangeably as if they meant the same thing or dealt with the same aspect of reality. At other times, we use them with a rigid compartmentalization and contribute to multiple reifications claiming exclusive priority in the explanation of an event.

Since there is no "real" or truly standardized definition of a variety of terms we will use, we take responsibility at this point for clarifying and distinguishing among certain terms.

Psychiatry.   This is a medical specialty whose central concern is the diagnosis and treatment of the sick and disturbed person (or more recently, family).

Social psychiatry.   In this branch of psychiatry, concepts and approaches from public health and sociology are used in an attempt to understand differences in incidence and prevalence of mental illness among various groups with respect to demographic and epidemiologic data. Examples include the high incidence of schizophrenia among lower class populations or the high incidence of suicide attempts among young adults between ages 18 and 25. A social psychiatrist can approach his therapy with a patient by taking into account particular social characteristics which specify that person in terms of age, sex, ethnic or racial group, and particular life circumstances. The term social psychiatry, like social medicine, is more English and European in use. Its less frequent use here may reflect political and economic attitudes against the word "social" being used in connection with any aspect of medicine.

Community psychiatry. This approach is less theoretical than social psychiatry. The term community psychiatry generally implies the application of psychiatric theories, skills, and procedures, particularly associated with social psychiatry, to the identification and treatment of disturbed persons as these are found in the community.

Mental health. Mental health refers to a state of psychosocial well-being, including those factors which promote and enhance it.

Community mental health. Again, this term relates to the more specific application of mental health principles to a defined population group. Practice within community mental health centers has emphasized the treatment of pathology, whether individual, family, or group. The enhancement and promotion of healthy adaptive behaviors in well and sick populations has been underestimated. Clinical treatment is the major event occurring within the walls of community mental health centers. For a community mental health center to become effective in the promotion of mental health and adaptation, its personnel and programs must move out of the clinic into the larger community, and work directly on the attitudes, behaviors, and processes within social institutions.

Although we have included a definition of community psychiatry, we are not particularly bound to it, and we have some definite reservations about the term. "Community" has become a mystical expression, laced with rhetoric, overloaded with symbolism, and charged with emotional connotations[21]. Promoters of community mental health centers said that they would make communities healthier. Critics and detractors took them at their word and then pointed to the failures. Urbanologists consider substandard housing, unemployment, rat infestation, and other poor conditions as indices of community ill health. They mentioned the social need for fraternal concern and commitment to mutual welfare among groups living in the same neighborhood, and then focused on alienation, apathy, and crime as reflections of community breakdown.

We eschew such an approach, and will not use "community" in any substantive or significant sense. Rather, from our vantage point as clinicians, we will talk about that which we know. We do know about mental health principles and practices, we can indentify populations at-risk, and we will discuss how we attempted to improve the lot of particular individual persons and groups within a community. What this does for the mental health of the "community" at large, we do not know nor care to speculate.

Table 1.1
Glossary of Terms: Reverent and Irreverent

Term	Explanation
Budget	A listing of priorities
Caretaker or caregiver	The one who is in the direct relationship of providing care or help to another.
Client	Patient
Consultation	I try to help you or your institution, or both, with a problem. I present some options to you; the responsibility for action remains yours.
Consumer	Client, patient, student, guest (also referred to as the overt consumer)
Hidden or covert consumer	The staff of a care-giving institution or other service institution
Diagnosis or labeling	It is done for several or all of the following reasons: 1. Medical and psychiatric tradition demands it 2. As a statistical device for research, administrative, and funding purposes 3. For the cognitive comfort of the diagnostician and his fellows 4. As a message that the diagnosee is a one-down position. Hence, this provides a one-up position for all others. This is an example of Stephen Potter's axiom: "If you're not one up, you're one down."[22] 5. For obfuscatory reasons 6. As a guide to treatment or helping activities, or both 7. As a device that says "You don't fit our school, our clinic, our program," and thus is used either to keep people out or to get them out. 8. As a way of saying, "This person is a bad apple."
Dirty work	That which we avoid and shift to someone else if we can.
Dirty workers	Those who care for the sick, handicapped, prisoners, the indigent, the very young and very old.[23]
Disturbed	Unhappy
A fox in the chicken coop	A very useful but difficult to implement strategy of introducing people who "don't belong there" into the innards of a social institution. Examples are paraprofessionals in professionally dominated institutions, parents in classrooms. The overt consumers become more intimately involved with the policies and practices of the institutions.

Table 1.1 *(Continued)*
Glossary of Terms: Reverent and Irreverent

Term	Explanation
	Also, as "flea in the shirt," the Russian version of fox in the chicken coop. (Acknowledgment to Mr. Khrushchev during his visit to the United States. When asked why there were no free elections in Russia, the irreverent chairman responded, "What man puts a flea in his shirt?")
Ham and eggs metaphor	As first heard from Dr. John Romano, this is an example of the double contingency paradigm. It reads "If we had ham, we could have ham and eggs, provided we had the eggs." This can be an early stage of the game, "Ain't it awful."
Innovative	New and good, as contrasted to just plain "new" which can be either good or bad
Intervention	You and I, separately or together, act on a problem.
Mainstream	The ordinary daily activities and situations that comprise the usual life experiences of people. For children, these center around the family, the school, the neighborhood, and the peer group.
Making it	Adapting: moving ahead in the personal, social, and cultural realm despite the stresses and restrictions of the environment
Mentally ill	Emotionally ill, emotionally disturbed, crazy, troubled, or troublesome
Relevant	Generally used in the context "not relevant," meaning what I'm doing is worthwhile; what you're doing isn't.
Retarded	Low IQ score. Also is used covertly to connote "Get him out of here."
Sideline	Being out of the mainstream, e.g., in a hospital, detention center, a clinic (even temporarily), a special class, a foster home
Sit lux erat lux (Genesis I:1)	And God said: "Let there be light and there was light." This metaphor alludes to the common practice of believing that the word is the deed. It is one of the many forms of magical thinking.
Snake oil	The universal remedy, solvent, and panacea for all problems and ailments. Mental health is often purveyed as one form of modern snake oil.
Status rub-off	The status of the client affects the status of the caregiver, e.g., psychiatrists working in state hospitals are viewed as inferior by their colleagues because their patients are seen as inferior by society.

REFERENCES

1. Report of the Joint Commission on Mental Health of Children. Crisis in Child Mental Health: Challenge for the 1970's. New York, Harper & Row, 1969

2. Group for the Advancement of Psychiatry. Crisis in child mental health: a critical assessment. New York, GAP Publication No. 82, 1972, p 111

3. Rosenthal D, Kety SS (eds): The Transmission of Schizophrenia. Oxford, Pergamon, 1968

4. Heston LL, Denney D: Interactions between early life experience and biological factors in schizophrenia. In Rosenthal D, Kety SS (eds): The Transmission of Schizophrenia. Oxford, Pergamon, 1968, pp. 363–376

5. Eysenck HJ (ed): Behavior Therapy and the Neuroses. New York, Macmillan, 1960

6. Alexander FG, Selesnick ST: The History of Psychiatry. New York, Harper & Row, 1966

7. Zilboorg G: A History of Medical Psychology. New York, Norton, 1941

8. Sullivan HS: The Interpersonal Theory of Psychiatry. New York, Norton, 1953

9. Spiegel J: Transactions: The Interplay Between Individual, Family and Society. New York, Science House, 1971

10. Berne E: Transactional Analysis in Psychotherapy: A Systematic Individual and Social Psychiatry. New York, Grove, 1961

11. Bowlby J: Attachment. New York, Basic Books, 1969

12. Tulkin SR, Kagan J: Mother-child interaction in the first year of life. Child Dev 43:31–41, 1972

13. Jackson DD: The study of the family. Family Process 4:1–20, 1965

14. Minuchin S, Montalvo B, Guerney BG Jr, Rosman BL, Shumer F: Families of the Slums. New York, Basic Books, 1967

15. Merton RK: Social Theory and Social Structure. New York, Free Press, 1957

16. Argyris C: Integrating the Individual and the Organization. New York, Wiley, 1964

17. Parsons T: The Social System. New York, Free Press, 1951

18. Pasamanick B, Knobloch H: Epidemiologic studies on the complications of pregnancy and the birth process. In Caplan G (ed): Prevention of Mental Disorders in Children. New York, Basic Books, 1961, pp 74–94

19. Spiegel, J: Transactions: The Interplay between Individual, Family and Society. New York, Science House

20. Jackson DD: The study of the family. Fam Process 4:1–20, 1965

21. Panzetta AF: Community Mental Health: Myth and Reality. Philadelphia, Lea and Febiger, 1971

22. Potter S: The Complete Upmanship. New York, Holt, 1971

23. Hughes E: Good people and dirty work. Soc Probl 10:3–11, 1962

Part I

Clinical Services

2

Metamorphosis of a "Traditional" Child Guidance Clinic into a Community Psychiatry Clinic

It is axiomatic to state that change is necessary for growth. It is equally trite and true that the ingredients for change may include mixes of fortune and deliberation, zeal and resistance, speed and delay. In retrospect, we seem rational experts about how changes occurred. While in the midst of change we are anxious, confused, pleased, or too often, oblivious.

One of the authors (M. Forman) has been associated with a child guidance clinic for 9 years; he began as a fellow in child psychiatry and is presently the clinic director. During that time, changes have occurred which appear to parallel events within the larger field of child psychiatry. Although our experience may be partly idiosyncratic, we share these reflections with you in the hope that our clinical impressions may be useful in the sense that if we know where we have been, we may have some idea of where we are going. (Hersch[1] gives an excellent description of modifications that are required in clinic function and structure to meet the needs of poor populations.)

The clinic which has undergone metamorphosis, or at least considerable change, is located in an "inner city," that is, a poor setting in metropolitan Philadelphia. It serves as the mental health outpatient unit of a pediatric hospital as well as the training section in child psychiatry for a medical school.

What changes have we faced? Who are we serving? How have we modified our approach? We examine two cases which illustrate changing times, populations, and problems. These two, one from 1964, and the other from 1968, were not chosen because they necessarily typify our patients. They were chosen because they underline the challenge to our clinic.

CASE 1

Date of Evaluation: 2/10/64

Tom W. is an 8-year-old boy, the oldest in a sibship of three. The children live with their parents, Herbert, age 40, and Miriam, 33. Father is a college graduate with a degree in accounting, and is currently employed as a sales manager for a large company. His work involves extensive traveling, and he may be home only 3 or 4 days a week. Mother, a housewife, is a high school graduate, with 2 years of business school training.

Tom was referred to the clinic by a private psychologist. The parents complained that their relationship with Tom was quite poor. They described him as being rebellious and quarrelsome at home, but without having any problems in school. At times, both parents felt that Tom's behavior was "impossible." Once father told Tom that they were going to send him to an orphanage. The parents then had to retract their statement after Tom struck back with an expressed desire to go to one. When his parents are having a discussion, Tom thinks that they are quarreling, and tells parents to get a divorce. He says that he will go with his mother. Mother finds Tom actually quite jealous of his father, but also admits that there are times when he seems closer to his father than he is to her. In describing Tom's personality, mother refers to him as a "cry baby" who is a "wise guy" and "often acts like he is an adult."

In discussing the marital situation, the parents admitted they were having problems with each other but claimed that Tom was the cause of their being "at each other's throats." Tom seemed able to behave in a way which antagonized the parents to the point that they were not able to deal with him or each other because of their own anger. They felt that Tom appreciated nothing that was given to him, despite receiving more than other children in the family.

The initial psychiatric evaluation of Tom revealed the diagnosis of psychoneurotic anxiety reaction, with the following comments on dynamics: "Tom is caught in an ongoing Oedipal struggle in which mother encourages his intellectual ability, his competition with father, and uses him as a neurotic substitute for father who is often physically absent from the house. Tom feels that too much is expected of him as an 8-year-old and that his parents have placed him in a bind: If he acts like a grown up, he will be given too much responsibility, but really will not be allowed to do what he wants. If he is a child, his needs will not be fulfilled because they were not fulfilled when he was much younger. Psychotherapy is indicated for Tom, but may be somewhat threatening for him because unconsciously he equates any freeing up of expression with a total loss of control in which he might display all of his anger. He seems to expect punishment from father, yet his major problems are related to mother. He seems to have an effectively implanted superego and to expect punishment for any stepping out of line. Parents will need considerable help in understanding their own unconscious behavior toward Tom, in addition to his own need for help with his internalized hostility."

For the next year and a half, parents were seen in counseling by a caseworker, and a child psychiatry resident carried on weekly psychotherapy with Tom.

Several joint sessions were also held with Tom, parents, caseworker, and resident. Father was seen at infrequent intervals because of his job situation, but mother and Tom did come for interviews on a weekly basis. As treatment progressed, there were some slight gains in insight. Mother became more aware of her anger toward her husband for his lack of emotional support and withdrawal; father acknowledged his tendency to withdraw, but also expressed a need for affection from his wife. Tom, however, remained uninvolved in the therapeutic process and demonstrated little change. The parents decided to terminate treatment, allegedly because of Tom's lack of progress but the caseworker felt that they were significantly threatened by some of the insights into their own behavior. At the time of termination, the caseworker and child psychiatry resident felt that relatively little had been accomplished in terms of changes in the family's feelings and behavior.

No formal follow-up has been obtained on this family, but it is known that Tom, at age 17, applied for outpatient psychiatric care at a local clinic.

CASE 2

Date of Evaluation: 1/5/68

Robert M., at the time of the original evaluation, was a 6.5-year-old first grade student, the second oldest in a sibship of five. Father, age 32, is a machine operator, and mother is a housewife. Robert was referred to the clinic at the suggestion of the school counselor who described him as "difficult to manage, having frequent temper tantrums, and screaming." Robert had been suspended from school over the Christmas holidays and school refused to readmit him until a psychiatric evaluation has been completed.

Parents denied having any problem with Robert at home and felt that the school counselor and principal were always blaming their son for things they felt he did not do. (Later they stated that the school personnel, who were white, showed prejudice toward black children). Mother, however, did indicate that she was having considerable difficulty with her husband, who admitted to being a heavy drinker. Mr. M. had had an almost nonexistent formal education but was able to advance in his job from sweeping floors to a semiskilled position. Mrs. M. has also worked periodically throughout the marriage and is currently employed in the housekeeping department of a local children's hospital. In spite of both parents' employment, the M. family has often faced financial crises, occasionally having had to move because of failure to pay rent. The intake worker recorded that Mrs. M. "seems to have little awareness of the children's needs and what is appropriate for them in order to grow up. Her handling of the children ranges from beating them in a fit of anger to being excessively permissive. Mr. M. is rarely at home in the evenings, and has little contact with the children." An initial home visit revealed a dismal and bleak home, with a dearth of facilities and furnishings.

Psychiatric evaluation of Robert viewed him as a "basically deprived child in a very unstimulating, impoverished homelife. Primary work with the family is needed, using a direct educative process to get this family going in a different direction. Robert has been handicapped by the deficiencies in his home situation so that he is unable to cope with his environment in a constructive way." Psychological testing revealed that Robert was presently functioning in the borderline retarded range, with a full scale IQ of 76. There was no evidence of any specific area of learning disability, but rather he seemed limited by a lack of healthy learning experiences.

A psychiatric social worker, who met the parents at the point of intake, then began working directly with the parents. After the evaluation was completed, she contacted a local school who agreed to readmit Robert while counseling with the parents went on. Mr. M., however, did not come to the appointments with his wife, so consequently a series of home visits were scheduled by the caseworker. Although Mr. M. agreed nominally to this agreement, he showed up for only part of one home visit, and consistently maintained that there was nothing he could do to help Robert. Robert was subsequently dropped from school again because of behavior difficulties in November 1968. He and his sister had been bussed to a new school after their old school had been torn down and he was unable to make the adjustment. The social worker kept working with Mrs. M., and also began including all the children in the sessions, both at home and in the office. Appointments, however, were kept infrequently, until Mrs. M. stated that she did not see the value of talking, since she had so many crises with which to cope. The social worker then moved from attempting to help Mrs. M. by counseling to direct work with the children and Mrs. M. together with the aim of stimulating their interest in learning. Family sessions became teaching sessions with the caseworker enlisting Mrs. M. as an ally in the process. The worker used several books, games, puzzles, and the alphabet to get the children moving. What became clear immediately was their tendency to become easily frustrated and to give up quickly, rather than persevering. The therapist was able to use this with Mrs. M. in helping her to see how frustrating school probably was for the children. Although Mrs. M. displayed some initial interest in this approach, once again attendance became irregular.

After accidentally meeting the social worker on the street, Mrs. M. came back a year later to discuss the possibility of separating from Mr. M. but then decided she could not do it. Robert had been back in school for about 6 months after mother had transferred him to another school which she felt was more cooperative.

Two years later, Mrs. M. again contacted the clinic, after Robert had been expelled once again. At this point, the psychiatric social worker asked for a consultation from a staff psychiatrist who saw Robert and placed him on medication. Mother felt that the family situation had been considerably improved and that her husband drank much less, was home more frequently, and getting along better with her. Robert maintained his improved state on medication for about 6 months, until another series of outbursts in school caused him to be expelled again. At this point, the social worker has referred Robert to a special day school for emotionally disturbed children operated jointly by the clinic and the public school system. Participation by the parents is mandatory in the program, and parents at least state at this point that they are willing to be involved to help Robert. Consideration has also been given to moving Robert away from home and placing him in a group foster home maintained by the clinic while he attends the day school program, but this option is being held in reserve until it is determined how Robert functions in the day treatment program.

Note that both cases have had relatively unsuccessful outcomes. Although the problems presented by Robert M. and family seem of greater intensity and may be more disabling in terms of impairment of school, work, and personal relationships, the myth has persisted that we accomplished more satisfactory results in the "old days" with "easier" and "better treatment" cases. Our task may have seemed easier, since we and our patients spoke a congruent middle class language, but measures of success were equally elusive then as now. Data from the literature certainly indicate that child psychotherapy is still an unproved treatment vehicle, regardless of the social class of the patient.[2] We should also emphasize that some of the techniques and suggestions used in case 2 could have been used in case 1. Home visits, family therapy, possible placement—all might have been quite appropriate for Tom and family. However, they were not tried, essentially because they were not the kinds of things mental health clinics did in 1964. More specifically, those also were not the methods that middle class therapists felt comfortable with when they dealt with middle class patients.

The two examples present marked differences in social class, source of referral, type of problem, diagnostic formulation, and services offered. In 1964, almost all of the clinic's patients came from outside the neighborhood, and were from white families of average income. Today, over 95 percent of our children come from the community, almost 50 percent from families on public assistance (the remainder with marginal incomes), and are of mixed racial and ethnic backgrounds. The effects of poverty, social disorganization, poor nutrition, and inadequate schooling on lower class children are well known, yet many survive because of coping skills that are less clearly understood. A significant question is how did we, as a clinic, use our adaptive skills to change and make our mental health interventions relevant to new needs and new populations. This does not imply that we have measured, or can measure, success objectively in terms of either prevention or treatment. But at least we are very busy; we feel that the community of patients and families want and need us; they have a reasonably low missed-appointment rate. We receive numerous requests for consultative programs; we are financially stable; we continue to attract trainees; and we have managed to survive, whereas several other similar local agencies have not. In 1964, we were a "traditional" child guidance clinic, analytically oriented, using long-term psychotherapy, and employing social workers, psychologists, and child psychiatrists in their classical diagnostic and therapeutic roles. In 1964, total staff complement was 12 with a budget of $125,000. In 1973, the clinic has a caseload almost exclusively from the community, offers brief therapy, family and group therapy, behavior modification, and chemotherapy, as well as individual psychotherapy; the clinic operates a day school program jointly with the school district for 40 severely emotionally disturbed children; it maintains a group foster home; it trains paraprofessionals; the clinic uses high school students as therapists; and it has supported numerous consultation programs in the community and adjacent pediatric hospital. The total paid staff number 35, with an annual budget of over $700,000.

The changes in the past decade cannot be attributed to a global deliberate design, but rather represent the coalescence of intuition, opportunism, commitment, and luck. We cannot reconstruct a meaningful chronology which demonstrates the sequence of change, but we do believe the change in our clinic was accomplished because, without always knowing it, we adhered to certain fundamental principles. Looking back, it appears that these were the guiding themes which assisted us.

"Tradition" Is Not Always Bad

The title of the chapter, "Metamorphosis of a 'Traditional' Child Guidance Clinic into a Community Psychiatry Clinic" can be taken to mean a change from "bad" to "good." Such is not our intent, however, and if we are misunderstood, it indicates the common cultural tendency to view old as bad, new as good, and "innovative" as best.

In our clinic, change came gradually in a program which had always stressed sound clinical experience, in-depth exploration of children and families, and thorough supervision. These are important virtues, regardless of theoretical orientation and no community psychiatry program should neglect them. Our clinic was not radically and suddenly changed; rather we built on our strengths and realized that our previous training in understanding individual psychodynamics was quite useful though not sufficient, as we extended our activities. As the social class of our patients changed, we did not attempt to fit them into the Procrustean bed of one particular theory of behavior, but we did try to understand their lives with the same degree of care and consideration we had used in the past. As we increased the extent of our services and made our interventions briefer and more directed, we continued to guard against superficial or slipshod work.

There were other clinic "traditions" which fostered our development. At a very personal level, there was an enduring sense of a staff "family" within the clinic. People cared for and liked each other. Often it appeared that it was a sense of commitment to each other and the program that kept us going, rather than any firm allegiance to an ideological notion. Staff had been, and continued to be involved in all phases of decision making, rather than serving as mere recipients of paternalistic edicts. This broad sharing of responsibilities often caused us to move slowly, but it also enabled us to "get it together" before we moved. Individual initiative and flexibility had always been valued. A staff member tells a seemingly trivial but quite significant story which typifies our tradition: He had asked his supervisor, a child analyst of rather conservative reputation, whether he should send Christmas cards to his patients, and they discussed the pros and cons. The supervisor encouraged him to experiment, to send cards to half his patients, using the other half as a control, and see the results for himself. The example reflected the notion that the patients will tell us if we can listen, and that we were also free to ask the questions. These values are our legacy from the past, and we hope that our future colleagues who will view us as "traditional," will also have that legacy from us.

Do Not Use Child Psychiatrists, Clinical Psychologists, and Psychiatric Social Workers in Their Usual Roles

In the historical child guidance approach, social workers saw parents and took histories, psychologists did testing, and the child psychiatrist interviewed the child. When the field was in its infancy, such a tripartite collaborative arrangement (or the "holy trinity" as Redl[3] called it) perhaps could be justified on the grounds that each discipline was finding its way and needed to develop its own professional identity and training program. By relying on the medical model, the division of labor also served the needs of the child psychiatric physician who was the leader of the team. The members of the other two disciplines provided him with extensive diagnostic information and made his own task easier.

As a clinic begins to see larger numbers of poor patients, the weaknesses of the traditional diagnostic method become apparent. Scheduling appointments with all these disciplines takes much time, and conferences must be arranged among the involved staff to collate the information gathered, which in some instances is of dubious reliability.[4] Families become confused about what is being done, they do not know who the primary caregiver is and may quickly and quietly drop out. Clinics can no longer afford the luxury of inefficient, protracted, data and wool gathering, while children and families need prompt and practical service.

In our clinic, we put into practice the logical assumption that experienced clinicians of whatever discipline possess skills that children and families need. As much as possible the family at the point of intake was assigned to *one* person—a child psychiatrist, psychologist, or social worker—who was responsible for diagnosis, planning, and implementation of appropriate treatment. Other staff members were called in to assist in the diagnostic or treatment process whenever their specific talents were required. Essentially the initial staff member serves as an expert in family management who may work with the total family, the parents only, the parents and the child separately, depending on the need. Other staff serve as consultants or cotherapists, on request. In a sense the more traditional idea of collaboration has persisted, but on a somewhat different, and more informal, basis. If a primary therapist for a child is required, a social worker or a psychologist can be just as competent as a child psychiatrist; if marital counseling is indicated, a child psychiatrist can do it, and a child psychiatric trainee should certainly gain experience with it. Personal talents and skills may be much more important than previous training.

Such "blurring" of disciplines presents problems, however. The boundaries are not totally erasible: the child psychiatrist, as a physician, is better equipped and socially sanctioned to deal with matters which involve organic illness and medication; a clinical psychologist knows how to administer and interpret psychological tests; a psychiatric social worker has the most experience with parents. Consequently, staff development is needed to update training in diagnostic and treatment techniques for persons whose previous experience has been narrow and limited. Resistance may flourish in all quarters. The child psychiatrist loses prestige if everyone else can do almost all that he has been so exclusively trained for. The psychologists had suspected this all along, but still want their own identity in order to maintain their influence with clinic administration. Social workers, as low persons on the totem pole, may feel that they are being asked to do most of the work for the least pay. Since we were an "old" clinic, changing to a different one, but without federal community mental health funding, we did not immediately confront the issue of a "new" discipline altogether, that is, that of the paraprofessional. Our task was not made easier by the lack of a paraprofessional challenge, however, since we all had to enlarge our own roles and competence, as we "blurred" the disciplines.

Do Not Separate Community Mental Health Services from Training Programs

Sections of child psychiatry and departments of general psychiatry have established separate, not always equal, programs in which service and training clinics are operated as different arms of the same organization. A typical model is one in which the service-giving staff, often using paraprofessionals, functions in a satellite neighborhood clinic or mental health center, whereas the training for child psychiatry residents and other disciplines occurs in a more academically oriented, more protected setting elsewhere in the parent institution. In the former location, patients with a variety of perplexing and discouraging problems of social disorganization are seen. In the latter, "appropriate training cases" are accepted, generally those manifesting a range of neuroses, or interesting character disorders deemed more suitable for insight-oriented psychotherapy. Such a "goats" versus "sheep" philosophy has been explicitly justified on the grounds that trainees learn better in a more structured setting where they can pick and choose a balanced caseload, and investigate their patients in some depth under the guidance of their supervisors. In the past, however, this dichotomous approach has often served to segregate patients more because of their social class and attractiveness than by any valid diagnostic criteria, with the more middle class clients being seen by the more middle class residents and supervisors.

This dualism is not only actually or potentially discriminating but also it just does not make sense when one is trying to administer an effective service and training operation. First, there is every reason to believe that there is a wide and varied range of psychopathology in lower social class patients, certainly more than enough to fill residents' needs. Moreover, the felt or imagined needs of residents should not be allowed to dictate the shape of the overall program. We viewed the training of residents as an important aspect of our clinic's function, but also emphasized training for psychology interns, social work students, medical students, and later, paraprofessional students. Second, if the problems of the lower class are more serious and complex, they should be treated in settings where the best supervision can be provided, not out in the "boon docks" far removed from the training program. If we feel that paraprofessionals can relate better in some instances to lower class patients, let us bring them and their patients both into the university departments where they may each have an impact on the institution. Third, there is a rather ubiquitous tendency to identify the status of caregivers with that of their clients. Therefore, within a school the teachers of retarded pupils often have the lowest status among their peers because of their rather nonglamourous work with their handicapped students, as compared to the more prestigious role of high school English teachers, for example. The psychiatrist who treats poor chronic schizophrenics in a state hospital system is a second class citizen compared to his analytic colleague who sees affluent neurotics. (See glossary, Table 1.1, the "status rub-off" effect.) In terms of the community service versus training dilemma, staff who are assigned to the "downtown" community clinic may be viewed as inferior to those who work in the more academic, "high falutin" program, as a social worker from another agency reported to us. And fourth, programs that continue to split training from community service may jeopardize their funding. As of this movement, psychiatry programs are being funded primarily with public monies, and governmental funding agencies are distinctly favoring service over training. If the amount of money expended for mental health programs should shrink further, it is logical to assume that the public agencies will be more interested in care for patients than in training of residents. Isolated training clinics, in which the patients serve as the grist for the trainee mill, will either accommodate or perish. Although confirmatory data would be impossible to get, our impression has been that psychiatric departments have a long history of diverting service funds to underwrite the inadequate subsidization of training costs. Such practices are more defensible, although still subject to criticism, in programs that offer training wholly within the context of services to the community. Then, at least, we are training persons who may ultimately be useful to the needs and interests of the local community.

Do Not Make a Commitment to Community Services Unless You Mean It

This sounds like a rather sophomoric admonition, comparable to telling a child to watch out for traffic before he crosses the street. We are elevating it to the status of a principle because we feel that it was often overlooked when organizations began receiving community mental health monies and yet continued to operate on a business-as-usual basis. Business-as-usual meant more of the same, traditional techniques applied to a few more poor people, numerous obstacles to service at the point of intake, exclusion of "organic" and retarded children from psychotherapy, lack of evening hours and emergency service, separate community versus training clinics, and an overall relegation of community needs to a second-level priority status. Obtaining public mental health funds to provide community services really means that a clinic has to *do* it, and not just *look* like it is doing it while it tries to do something else; for example, using community funds to hire junior staff members whose primary function is teaching. Clinics can be, and have been, caught by their communities and their funding services. Some have even gone out of business. In a sense, a clinic is in the service business, and ideally there should be a proper fit between what the consumer wants and what the clinic can provide. We have not achieved truth-in-packaging since we do not know specifically what are the best kinds of mental health services or how they can be most adequately delivered, but let us at least be clear with our public that we are searching with them and not using their money to further our own institutional aims.

Extend the Definition of "Treatment"

What is treatment? Is it a child psychiatrist doing long-term insight psychotherapy with an obsessive compulsive girl? A black high school student teaching basketball to an 8-year-old fatherless black boy? A mental health counselor from the community illustrating techniques of limit setting to a family? A contract between a social worker and a mother for six sessions to work on the problem of an impending divorce and its impact on the family? A series of discussions on child-rearing principles with emphasis on direct advice giving, conducted by a clinical psychologist? A behavior modification program for an 11-year-old boy with enuresis? A tutorial program organized by a special education consultant for a group of clinic patients and their siblings? The use of stimulant medication for a first grader with hyperactivity? The participation of psychiatrists on a renal dialysis team to assist the nursing and medical staff in their work with patients and with their own feelings?

We suggest that it is all of these and that a clinic must offer a variety of approaches to children and families who have a variety of problems. Too long has "treatment" been viewed as a kind of sanctified method growing out of a rigid ideological belief.[5] The word "treatment" has generally been used in a medical context, but it has other meanings, as well. For instance, the dictionary definition of the word "to treat" includes the following:[6]

1. To act or behave toward (a person) in some specific way: *to treat someone with respect;*
2. To consider or regard in a specific way, deal with accordingly;
3. To deal with (a disease, patient, etc.) in order to relieve or cure, as a physician does;
4. To deal with in speech or writing; discuss;
5. To deal with, develop, or represent artistically, especially in some specified manner or style: *to treat a theme realistically;*
6. To subject to some agent or action in order to bring about a particular result;
7. To entertain; to give hospitality to;
8. To carry on negotiations with a view toward settlement; discuss terms of settlement.

All definitions are appropriate in a mental health setting since all are relevant to the human condition. In broadening the definition beyond its usual medical-psychiatric connotation (number 3, above) we also recognize that nonmedical personnel can do "treatment" and really have been doing it all along. Their treatment efficiency may depend much more on their skills related to the eight definitions listed above than on any previous medical-psychiatric training. Even in a sound medical approach, we would agree that first one should determine what the patient needs, and then who is the best person to render it. Too often in the past, we have attempted to use one particular kind of service giver, offering one specific type of service.

Organize the Staff into Service Teams

As our clinic moved toward offering more community services, we accepted the responsibility for the mental health care of children and families living within two specific, but rather large catchment areas. These catchment areas, lying on either side of the clinic, contain dissimilar populations, but who often manifest similar problems. One area is about 80 percent black, with a large number of single-parent families on public assistance and a high degree of mobility. The other is over 90 percent white, representing predominantly blue collar, two-parent families with firm generational ties within the neighborhood. Both sections have comparably high degrees of social disintegration, as reflected in rates for alcoholism, drug abuse, juvenile delinquency, imprisonment, and state hospitalization. In addition to providing services to these two areas, we are also involved in giving care and consultation to children referred from the inpatient and outpatient medical services of our pediatric hospital.

To allow for a maximum of flexibility and intensity in response to these service demands, we organized our services into three teams, one for each area (the two communities and the hospital). The teams were composed of staff and trainees in the various disciplines, and they functioned essentially as semiautonomous miniclinics. They handle the intake from each area, assign cases to their members, are forced to struggle with devising new approaches to deal with large numbers of patients, respond to local community requests for program consultation and planning, offer orientation courses for school counselors, assist the pediatricians, and have many informal contacts with other human service givers in the community and hospital. Within a team, no separation was made between "direct service" and "indirect service" (program consultation). Team members participated in both, using their clinical skills as a basis for working with other caretaking personnel (pediatricians, teachers, counselors, and others) in order to enhance their efforts with children and families. Referring agents in the community and hospital deal with an identifiable and visible group within the clinic rather than a number of disparate persons. The team gets to know the community, whether it be a neighborhood or hospital, and the community or at least segments within it get to know the team. Such relationships offer opportunities for effective liaison programs and bridge building involving clinic, families, and social institutions.

The team structure also offers a fair measure of support to staff who are immersed in the sorting out of difficult problems in mental health care. Team members can use each other for assistance and consultation, bring problems to team meetings, and learn from the skills of other members. On the negative side, team structure may also foster a spirit of competition within the clinic in terms of which team is the "best," but we should also note that one team may become resentful of another if it feels that the latter is doing "easier" work or is favored by the administration. A tendency to racial exclusivity of teams may occur in terms of black patients being seen by black staff on one team, whereas whites see whites on another. Each team should have a racially integrated staff, and have some experience, even on a limited basis, with patients from the opposite catchment areas who are from different racial backgrounds.

Involve the Administrator in Clinical Matters

The business administrator of our clinic happened to be a person who possessed extraordinary skills of financial management. Her abilities, however, could be exercised to the fullest extent because she was intimately familiar with our clinical activities. We know that mental health personnel generally have little or no background in business administration, and yet they are often in an unenlightened position of wanting to run programs without being "contaminated" by financial considerations. An effective administrator who participates in clinical meetings, who knows the working difficulties of staff and the sociopsychological problems of families can suggest strategies, maneuvers, and devices which may be able to secure or divert funds. Our administrator was particularly valuable in obtaining funding from local sources through effective politicking with county agencies, while the senior clinicians fretted more about federal funding which turned out to be of lesser importance. She was able to argue and lobby for us because she fully knew our program and could adequately articulate our needs as well as those of the patients we served. And, not to be overlooked, as a "layman," she added a note of practical sobriety to our more utopian dissertations and reminded us of what was workable and possible in this—not the best—of all possible worlds.

Be Initiators, Not Victims

We went through a difficult period in our clinic 5 years ago when it seemed as though the gods were angry and had conspired to work some magic against us. A series of events culminated in our feeling like passive victims who no longer had control over our fates. The clinic director, a much respected veteran teacher and clinician, had left for another position; our chief social worker, essentially the administrative cement of our operation, died. The state and federal governments, through their allocation of funds, were giving us as well as other clinics the message that we had to change our programs and yet the direction of change seemed uncertain. Our previous traditional training and service functions to a middle class population had been definite and orderly. Now both were receiving external challenges and internal questioning.

As in patients who are depressed, we temporarily retreated to a position of passivity and helplessness, wanting to maintain the old world and afraid of the new. The turning point, if one can truly be identified, occurred when the interim director decided to take advantage of some United Fund money to hire a community organizer. We could at least learn about our neighborhood, its schools, its problems, and its people. Perhaps, we and they could survive together. We began acting, rather than anticipating, and the activity, not always well planned and executed, served as a remedy. As we talked to local groups and agencies, it appeared that they needed our help. As we ventured outside clinic walls, the staff saw that perhaps we could change our attitudes and methods without severe disruption. Although our newer techniques and approaches still did not offer us the security and conceptual clarity of the old, at least we were doing something and becoming very busy in doing it. And out of shared doubts, frustration, and enthusiasm came a realization that we had managed to pull through and we had done it mostly by ourselves.

As we look over the above principles, they seem to err in the direction of appearing too deliberate and rational. We did not document all of our blunders, some of which have been thankfully forgotten. Nor have we given ample credit to luck. And, as in most endeavors, our hindsight now is better than our insight then.

REFERENCES

1. Hersch C: Child guidance services to the poor. J Am Acad Child Psychiatry 7:223–241, 1968
2. Levitt EE, Beiser, HR, Robertson RE: A follow-up evaluation of cases treated

at a community child guidance clinic. Am J Orthopsychiatry 29:337–349, 1959

3. Redl F: Crisis in the children's field. Am J Orthopsychiatry 32:759–780, 1962
4. Wenar C: The reliability of developmental histories. Psychosom Med 25:505–509, 1963
5. Gould RD: Dr. Strangeclass: or how I stopped worrying about the theory and began treating the blue-collar worker. Am J Orthopsychiatry 37:78–86, 1967
6. The Random House Dictionary of the English Language, College Edition, 1968

3

Development of a Children and Family Unit in a Community Mental Health Center

In 1966, the Department of Psychiatry of Temple University in North Philadelphia began planning for a community mental health center and hired a director to develop the program.* The mental health center was established as one of the major divisions of the department, coequal with the other major divisions, such as the inpatient and outpatient services. The director (Dr. Elmer A. Gardner) invited several other psychiatrists, psychologists, and other personnel to form the nucleus of the administrative and clinical sections of the mental health center. The first year was spent in planning and developing the mental health center grant application to be submitted to the federal government for funding (E. A. Gardner, unpublished, 1966).

The director and his unit chiefs shared a common belief that there was a need for more effective, available, and comprehensive services to the population for which the mental health center was responsible. The catchment-area population approximated 220,000 (1960 census): 80 percent black, with a median education of eighth grade, and a median income of $4,500. Unemployment was high and housing often inadequate. High infant and maternal mortality, short life expectancy, school dropouts, and delinquency substantiated the picture of a population in the grip of severe poverty.

*In 1973, as a result of negotiations with officials of the university and federal, state, and local governments, complete responsibility for the mental health center was transferred to a non-profit community group. The center was renamed North Central Philadelphia Community Mental Health and Mental Retardation Center.

In the early planning and development of the center, those persons who were heads of service units wrote a series of position papers, which outlined the objectives, methods, and functions of each of the service units. These papers were circulated and then discussed among the various unit chiefs as well as among other members of the staff. Questions, objections, criticisms, and problems of implementation were raised in these discussions. Central problems that required repeated attention not only in the planning stage, but after the center was in operation, included the interconnection of services and the relationship of units in terms of the integration of individual service goals, policies, and procedures with the overall goals, purposes, functions, and responsibilities of the mental health center. Ultimately, a contract of a verbal sort was negotiated between the director of the center and the various service chiefs and among each service as to how the units would operate, how they would work together to function as a whole. Such a contract is not one that is established once and for all, but one that is continually undergoing questioning and modification and revision. Conscious awareness of this fact and attention to this process is required in the light of the development of new needs and demands by the client population, changes in the staffing pattern of the center, and the requirements of the regulations of federal, state, and local legislative and administrative bodies.

The main administrative and outpatient units of the mental health center were located in a series of refurbished rowhouses scattered within a block or two of each other and approximately the same distance from the medical center hospital. The acute adult inpatient inservice was located in the university hospital, and the longer term inpatient service was located at a state hospital 15 miles away.

The psychosocial clinic was the major outpatient service. The crisis center (24-hr emergency service) and the psychosocial clinic were the two "service entrances" to the community mental health center. The rest of the service units were reached by a first stop in either the crisis center or psychosocial clinic. The front line, or direct access units, provided evaluation and treatment but also made triage decisions for patients in need of other services available in the mental health center: total hospitalization, partial hospitalization, rehabilitative, and vocational services. Particular relationships of the Children and Family Unit to the crisis center and psychosocial clinic will be made clear as we describe the development and operation of this unit. The development of the mental health center is described in several publications, and the problems involved in implementing the concepts of community mental health within the framework of the federal legislation are reviewed.[1−3]

One of the major innovations initiated and developed by Dr. Gardner was the mental health assistant training program.[3] Mental health assistants were new paraprofessional personnel trained within the center to be employed in each of the units of the center according to the needs and purposes of that unit. The mental health assistants served as a primary case manager and therapist in the psychosocial clinic. In the inpatient service, they functioned as group therapists and in the partial hospitalization service, they functioned as members of the staff of the therapeutic community approach. Other mental health assistants worked closely with community groups and organizations through the consultation and education unit. Here, we will briefly describe the function of the mental health assistants in the Children and Family Unit (see Chapter 10 for detailed description).

Implied in the whole concept of paraprofessional training and utilization was a redefinition of professional role, both generally and specifically. The major determinant of professional behavior is the discipline in which one is trained. In the community mental health center, the effect of professional discipline was diluted and modified by the additional factors of interest, skill, and initiative in the determination of job activities. Necessarily, certain essentials of the discipline were maintained, such as the physician's responsibility and exclusive prerogative for dealing with medication or recognizing and responding to the impact of physical disease on a person. Psychologists retained the role test administration and interpretation, but in the Children and Family Unit, took on significant treatment, supervisory, and consulting activities. In Chapter 10, there is a more detailed discussion of the problems related to the development of new roles and the changing of established ones.

PUTTING CHILDREN IN THEIR PLACE

Past practice has resulted in children and services to children receiving last consideration. Departments of psychiatry, mirroring the rest of society, believe in children and child psychiatry. Although the belief may be strongly asserted, children are, in fact, weak and small. Therefore, allocation of money, space, personnel, and program development to children's services is generally congruent with the size and strength of the client population.

The community mental health center legislation required that all five essential services be available and provide service to anyone in need in the catchment area.[4] This implicitly includes children. In fact, the reality of the mental health center's development has been quite negligent toward children. Children and services for them had been given a low priority.[5-7]

The results of a recently completed national survey of mental health centers conducted by Glasscote, Fishman, and Sonis revealed only a few centers where children's services were given priority and none where comprehensive services were in effect.[8] In the last 3 years there has been an attempt to rectify this neglect of children at the federal and local levels. The director of the National Institute of Mental Health has stated repeatedly that children are the first priority for mental health service. However, in fact, in these last 2 years of federal legislation, only 10 million dollars per year has been allocated for these "first priority" services, and presently the federal stream has run dry. At the time of this writing, the record and results at the local level have been worse.

In order to demonstrate concretely from the beginning the importance of children, it was essential to establish the Children and Family Unit as a separate administrative entity, coequal with the other "five essential service units." This meant the director of the Children and Family Unit (W. Hetznecker) was a member of the administrative planning and policy-making group of the mental health center.

A preeminent issue any administrator has to determine in developing a new program is the degree of his own autonomy. The director of the Children and Family Unit had considerable autonomy. After completing the planning process described above, each unit chief in the mental health center was free to develop his unit in the way appropriate to the reality of the needs of the population, the basic nature of the service, the kind and amount of staff available, and the restrictions of money and space. Such development took place within the frequently changing and often ambiguous guidelines of the federal and state regulations.

Conceptually, we believed that advocacy for children and their families was part of the mission of the Children and Family Unit. It was important to express this advocacy within the structure of the mental health center as well as to other agencies such as schools, courts, and health and welfare institutions which are responsible for children. To express this policy, in practice, required that the Children and Family Unit have administrative recognition within the center equal to the other services.

PRACTICES TO AVOID

At the level of practice, it is important to deal not only with what we wanted to do but also with what we wanted to avoid. We were concerned with responding realistically to present realities, in terms of concepts and practical methods of implementing these concepts, but we wanted to avoid those aspects of past practice that were not useful, again either at the level of either theory or practice. Some of these past practices are listed:

1. We wanted to avoid both the low status of children's services and the lack of influence they exerted.
2. We wanted to avoid the past practice that children's services had employed many professionals serving relatively few patients. The staff-client ratio in outpatient services was typically fairly high. There were, in addition, long waiting lists and many clinics excluded the sickest children with a tendency to provide treatment for those who were less disturbed or who were "good treatment" cases. The latter quality was determined according to particular psychotherapeutic beliefs held by the staff of the clinic. Time and people were not used economically in a triage system that tended to treat those with mild or moderate disturbances.
3. We wanted to avoid a reflex adherence to a status system of treatment modalities. Historically, one-to-one psychotherapy, preferably long term and analytically oriented, has been a high status treatment modality for children. This type of treatment was often used in many clinics as a vehicle for the training function. Cases of children to be treated were often picked with this dual function in mind. Frequently, the training function prevailed as an implicit criteria for acceptance. Implicitly, this also represented a classist policy with many clinics serving children from middle class and upper middle class backgrounds who were considered more appropriate for the preferred treatment modality. This practice was enhanced by certain exclusion criteria around such diagnostic entities as organic brain diseases, borderline mental retardation, or the use of such notions as lack of motivation on the part of poor families to become involved in treatment.[9-11] This practice also fostered an uneconomic use of time and people, and the result was that most expensive sort of treatment in terms of time, people, and cost was carried out first, last and always.
4. Another more nebulous, but real, practice we wished to avoid can be formulated: Only the "anointed" can touch the sick child and then each "anointed" only in certain ways. Such a formulation refers to the rigidly defined roles that existed in many child guidance clinics for each of the professional groups: psychiatrists, psychologists, and social workers. These restrictions not only produced an underutilization of the skills and knowledge of the various professionals but also excluded many other kinds of workers who could be useful in helping children. Such an approach tended to maintain the high status and administrative dominance of psychiatrists and buttressed the view that the medical model was the only way of looking at and dealing with mental or emotional disturbance.

5. We wanted to avoid an overemphasis on pathology, sickness, and maladaptation. Psychiatry, particularly clinical psychiatry, treats "sick," disturbed, ill people. As we stated in the first chapter, in addition to this basic and necessary function of treating the sick and disturbed, a mental health center should also find ways of identifying, promoting, and eliciting healthy coping behavior in persons, families, and social institutions. The primary role of our consultative interventions which will be described below was to promote adaptation between children and their various environments.

6. We wanted to avoid the fragmented service to adults and children which had existed in the past. Child guidance clinics see children as the primary patient and the parent is worked with as a collateral in terms of advice, guidance, and helping him understand his difficulties in relation to his child. Parental counseling is directed and oriented around the primary treatment of the child. If the adult happens to be defined as disturbed or in other ways in need of primary help, he or she is frequently referred to an adult hospital, clinic, or practitioner. The recent development of family therapy on an outpatient basis conceptualizes the family as the disturbed entity with the referred person as the symptomatic member or index of multiply disturbed relationships in family structure and organization. It is only within the last decade that this concept has been more generally applied to families of younger children and families whose index member is non-schizophrenic. Now many clinics and individual therapists emphasize the treatment of the whole family.[12-14] We believed that the mental health center should operate with a one-door policy so that children would not be entering one door to see one group of people and adults in the same family entering another door to be treated by another group of people.

7. We wanted to avoid the dumping or slough-off approach which occurs when people who are not trained as child specialists say, "I can't treat kids, I'm not trained. I don't know what to do." Then by reason of indifference and anxiety or unwillingness to get involved with children, they send a child to the child specialist. This attitude is justified through use of "only the anointed" theorem. Many who revert to this position when confronted with a disturbed child are the same people who deal with children in a variety of roles quite successfully and competently as parents, aunts, uncles, and in recreational, church, and other settings. Once the child is identified as "disturbed" or "sick" or "emotionally ill," the reaction is to avoid him. This is also one of the specific manifestations of the basic antichild attitudes existent in the culture (see Chapter 1). Underlying this attitude is some hostility and resentment toward children which might be formulated as follows:

"He's got a lot of nerve to get sick or be disturbed and expect me to do something about it." Another underlying feeling is anxiety generated by an unexpressed fantasy that the sick child is fragile or dangerous. There is a complementary fantasy that the adult is perhaps dangerous and capable of harming or making the child worse unless he is specially skilled or trained. This latter notion is connected with the general, more explicit idea that mental health disciplines have communicated and which unfortunately has been believed—that the sick child is the "victim" of the noxious actions and agency of adults, primarily the parent.

NEW AND REALISTIC POLICIES

Our approach to the organization of delivery of services was to call into question and examine each of these past practices in terms of the present realities. First, we recognized that a large number of primary caregivers and caretakers in the widest possible sense of parents, teachers, recreation workers, older teenagers are involved in helping relationships with healthy and distressed children. Second, we recognized that for the forseeable future, there will be an acute and chronic shortage of highly trained professional caregivers in the mental health field.[15] We further believed that the skills in being helpful to children can be improved in some, elicited and developed in others, and supported in still others. We concluded that one of our basic policies was to find ways to train, develop, elicit, and promote the helping skills of those primary caregivers who work with children in a variety of situations.

Within the direct operations of the mental health center and the activities of our unit, this approach was formulated into a policy. We saw ourselves as the child specialists who were more skilled and highly trained in the assessment of children's disorders. We saw our primary role then as being one of teaching and training of others in their direct work with children. Consequently, we initially established our unit as a backup service, not as a primary front line service. Children and adults came into the center through the psychosocial clinic or crisis center doorways. We served as backup personnel to the efforts of the generalists in the psychosocial clinic who were the primary caregivers of outpatient service. The tasks of our unit staff involved consultation, evaluation, and advice in the planning, management and treatment of children and families. Only in certain cases did we take over the direct management of child or family from the primary therapist. This latter decision was made on the basis of the seriousness of the disturbance of the child or family, and thus the need that the child specialist be directly involved in the service. As the unit grew larger and staff expanded, we saw that our direct service function would increase. This direct service aspect became more important when the mental health center became responsible for service to the mentally retarded as required under Pennsylvania legislation of 1966 and implemented in 1969.

Because of the multiple and complex problems that families with moderately and severely retarded children present, we later augmented staff capacity to provide direct services to these clients. The mildly retarded and those classified as borderline had from the beginning made up a fair portion of the client population of our mental health center. The initial service to this group was provided by the psychosocial clinic with the Children and Family Unit providing the backup support described above.

THE PROCESS*

To enhance the skills of the primary therapists, we relied heavily on the vehicle of the case-evaluation consultative interview. For example, in those instances in which a child was the primary client for service, after the first or any other visit, the primary therapist, whether paraprofessional or professional, could request consultative help from the staff of the Children and Family Unit. The consultation request was made on a simple form which identified the child, his age, his family composition, the school he attended, and a brief statement of the nature of his problem on admission. In addition, there was a statement by the consultee as to the questions or problems that he wished the consultant to be concerned with. Finally, there was a statement as to the present treatment or management procedure being carried out by the primary therapist.

The consultative appointment was arranged by the primary therapist. The mother, and on rare occasions the father, the index child, and frequently the other siblings were invited to come to the center. The primary therapist had previously explained that the child specialist would be talking with the child and parent. Prior to the time of the interview, the child specialist and primary therapist as well as the therapist's supervisor met to discuss the consultation request. At this meeting, the group reviewed any developments that had intervened between the request and the present appointment. The main purpose of the preliminary meeting was to identify the focus of the consultation interview, its aims, and goals. This was an essential part of the teaching-training task carried out by our unit's staff.

The interview was conducted by the consultant with the primary

---

*Marge Eckert, senior social worker, served as clinical coordinator of the Children and Family Unit, and facilitated the success of the consultative-training method by her sensitive liaison work with other units.

therapist and supervisor present. The initial part of the interview was held
with the parent and child together and in the latter part of the interview,
each family member was seen individually. The primary therapist and his
or her supervisor were present throughout. Note that no one-way screen or
mirror was available in the mental health center for these interviews. They
were conducted in a large room which served originally as an upstairs
bedroom in a rowhouse. The room was large enough so that four or five
people could be comfortable and allow enough distance between them.
Crowding and restriction of activity, especially for the children, was not a
problem.

The focus of the interview was determined by the nature of the
problem and to a large degree by the particular questions raised by the
primary therapist. The most common questions concerned diagnosis,
severity of problem, relationship between child and parent, or siblings, or
both, the child's attitude toward himself or school, and the child's intellectual capacity. Other questions concerned management approaches:
whether the child himself needed direct service, whether service should be
carried out with or through the agency of the parents, or primarily through
school personnel. Other questions concerned the degree to which all family
members, especially siblings should be involved in the treatment process.
An important issue that often required clarification was the nature of the
relationships of the particular family with other service agencies such as
welfare, family service, recreational, or other community groups. Questions about the indications for and the use of medication frequently arose.
As the primary therapist become more comfortable and sophisticated in
working with children, she became interested in discussing such issues as
the parents' divorce or separation and its effect on the children, the indications for and possible effect of placement of the child outside the home,
helping a child with his grief, and the feelings a child might have about
school failure or being placed in a special class. After the primary therapist
became comfortable with the consultative approach and trusting of the
consultant, she raised questions about her feelings and reactions to the
child and family. In helping resolve these issues some barriers to the
therapist's own effectiveness in working with a child or family became
manifest. Thus, the consultative approach was consultee centered as well
as client centered. To be effective in this consultative-training effort, it
was essential for the child specialist to have this in vivo experience jointly
with the family and the primary therapist. After concluding with the interview, the child specialist and primary therapist would discuss their observations and exchange ideas. The child specialist tried to focus on those
questions and issues raised by the primary therapist and introduced other
observations or inferences he might have made as he judged these to be

important in the overall work with the child and his family. The parents and child or children were then called back to the interviewing room and the child specialist summed up for them his findings and thoughts about the situation. He constantly referred to and included the primary therapist in any discussion of future planning. In whatever way possible, the child specialist supported, encouraged, and maintained the relationship of the child and his parent to the primary therapist. Even if there were a decision that the child and family specialist was to take over the direct care of the client, this decision was not communicated at the end of the initial consultative interview. Instead, the primary therapist would meet with the child and his family in the future for further planning and discussion of treatment approaches.

After the family had left, the child specialist had a more extended discussion with the primary therapist and supervisor present concerning his impressions and findings. Resorting to jargon frequently elicited the question from the primary therapist, "What do you mean by that?" and "How do I do that?" This kind of questioning, especially from paraprofessionals, kept professionals honest and freed them from the highly practiced skill of obfuscation. There are many reasons for using child specialists in this manner. First of all, we wanted to maximize our impact in terms of training through the use of modeling. We wanted to share some of the same data with the primary therapist. We wanted to help the consultee to focus and clarify issues through the requirement of a consultative request form and in the pre- and postevaluation discussions. In terms of modeling, we talked a good deal about interviewing technique after each interview. We talked about why we had asked certain questions and why we did not ask others. We stressed the joint interview of parent and child as showing us how people do business with each other. Another advantage of the joint interview of parent and child was to help overcome a tendency of any therapist to overidentify with one side or the other in the common generational disputes occurring in children and families. We constantly emphasized focusing on definable issues the child, parent, and therapist could understand and agree on. We continually used the terms *contract, deal,* or *bargain.* We wanted the therapist to learn to identify those contracts that were causing problems between the child and his parent or between the child and the school or among other family members. Further, we wanted to help identify those particular issues or problems that the child or family were willing to work on through a contract with the therapist.

The therapist who is inexperienced in working with children and families whether he be professional or paraprofessional, can frequently have trouble with two concepts: first, defining and focusing on issues, and second, working on realizable goals. One of the most common responses when dealing with clients from poverty areas who are experiencing multiple distresses at the environmental, social, intrafamilial, and intrapsychic levels is for the therapist to declare that the client is overwhelmed and for the therapist himself to share in that sense of powerlessness and feel overwhelmed also. One of the major values we held in therapy was that clients, and particularly children, needed to acquire some sense of competence, effectiveness, and mastery of those aspects of life over which it was reasonable and appropriate to have control. Reciprocally, we wanted to decrease the feelings of passivity, helplessness, and ineffectiveness as well as diminish those behaviors that were threatening and dangerous to others or themselves and which resulted in ineffective attempts at mastery and coping.[16] Since this was one of the major values and goals that we had for clients, it was naturally an important goal for therapists to have for themselves in their therapeutic work. An overwhelmed, helpless, passive therapist who sees himself unable to do anything about the terrible problems that beset his client is by reason of his own psychic stance unable to help that client develop effective coping strategies of self-determination.

We wished also to promote the enhancement of the client's self-esteem and self-respect and by extension, his respect and esteem for others. We felt that it was our job as consultants, models, and teachers to help the primary therapist maintain his own self-esteem of his therapeutic efforts. Our messages strongly emphasized the positive in what primary therapists were doing. We encouraged the employment and development of their natural tendencies, abilities, and skills. A third principle that we taught to nonchild specialists and implemented in our own approach to intervention was the concept of helping people "make it." We felt one of the most important things we could do was to help promote and encourage useful functioning in the various spheres of the child and family. This meant we were interested practically in the child and his mother and father making it together in terms of their day-to-day behaviors and interactions. We were interested in enhancing and promoting the child's making it in school academically and behaviorally. We wanted to help the child make it with his peers and most importantly, with himself. Function became a primary criterion by which we judged our therapy as useful or successful, and whether it should be terminated or continued.

In helping a child "make it" in school, we may be criticized for promoting conformity to a bad system. Our experience of 5 years demonstrates the limits of mental health centers in their programs to change "systems." It is important to point out the dangers inherent in using the client's nonconformity or otherwise retaliation-provoking behavior as a possible means of acting out the therapist's fantasies and wishes for changing or challenging the system. Changing the system does not come about by encouraging or promoting disruption of classrooms by children. This only promotes helplessness, anger, and retaliation on the part of teachers and the child suffers. If the mental health workers are only seen as siding with the child's negative behavior against the "bad system" or "bad adults," it will ultimately lead to the exclusion and isolation of mental health workers from the school or other institutions. The staff of such institutions will see mental health workers as being ineffective, useless, and possibly harmful. The institution of social change is clearly needed. Such change is clearly not effectively carried out by the mental health worker using the disturbing behavior of children as either evidence for the need for change or as an instrument to bring about such change.

We invoked the principle of parsimony: trying the simple, cheaper less technical approach before we tried the more expensive approach in terms of time and people. Practically, this meant that if we could persuade the school to change a child from one class to another and his disruptive behavior stopped, we felt this was enough intervention and no further help was needed at that moment. A second level of intervention might include advice to the teacher and the family and the use of reinforcement techniques: ignoring negative behavior, the judicious use of positive rewards in dealing with negativism, temper tantrums, or inattention in school. If the primary caretakers could effectively use these techniques after some periods of instruction, we considered the intervention sufficient and would leave the family system alone until they or the school requested help again. Long-term individual therapy with children or families was far down on the list of pertinent choices and was invoked after other interventions seemed to be fruitless and ineffective. We believed and promoted the approach that if a child could go to a recreation center and learn a skill or sport that increased his self-esteem, there would be no need for him to go to a clinic to talk to somebody about his poor self-esteem unless we could determine that there were additional benefits to derive from a relationship with a sympathetic and understanding adult in the clinical situation.

In our work with primary therapists, we eliminated emphasis on the hour therapy session. We encouraged therapists to see a child, parent, or family for as long as it seemed useful and useable, for both client and therapist. Frequently, patients were seen for an hour and even longer when home visits were made. In our teaching and training in the consultative sessions, we encouraged the therapist to use his own judgement as to the appropriate amount of time provided for any client at any session. Sessions then could vary in their duration from week to week or visit to visit.

EXTRAMURAL FUNCTIONS

We determined that the Children and Family Unit would be the main consultation and education group for agencies, institutions, and groups serving children as primary clients. We served this function to provide greater continuity of service, to be effective advocates for children outside the center, and to be certain that child-serving institutions were not neglected by our center programs or lost in the usual crunch of priorities. The Children and Family Unit had responsibility for what in other centers was carried out by the consultation and education unit under more general consultative responsibilities. The consultation and education unit at Temple consulted with the police department, the public health department, conducted seminar training programs in mental health for employees of various agencies, and provided field placement for seminary students. In many centers, it has been the practice for the consultation and education unit to be consultants for schools, juvenile courts, Get Set programs, day care centers, and welfare programs, as well as a variety of agencies which serve adults. As a consequence of such competing priorities, children frequently lose. In addition, the reality is that children who are clients of the various child service agencies are more at-risk than adults for being extruded out of the mainstream of life into sideline systems, especially mental health systems.

We wanted to avoid such past practices and to increase continuity of service between referring agencies and the center. Most important, we wanted to ensure and enhance the capacity of primary child care institutions to cope with children within their walls, by using all their resources. The primary institutions we related to were schools. We were also involved with preschool programs, welfare, and in a limited way, the courts. In succeeding chapters, we will describe certain programs that were developed with these institutions.

FORMAL TRAINING ACTIVITIES

In addition to the consultative and evaluative interviews we described, the staff of the Children and Family Unit carried out various formal training activities for other staff members of the mental health center. These included seminars on family therapy, discussions of diagnostic considerations of children and families, lectures in child development, the use and abuse of psychological tests, and case conferences related to treatment and management. These formal training sessions were at times directed primarily to paraprofessionals and other times to professional groups.

STAFFING

The unit was established with two professionals, a child psychiatrist, and a clinical psychologist. The psychologist, although initially inexperienced with children, availed herself of the opportunity to take advantage of the clinical interview training model described. Within a short time, she developed her skills at child and family interviewing so that she was able to double the clinical consulting and training resources of the unit.

Within the year, the staff of the Children and Family Unit was increased by the addition of a public health nurse, a social worker, a part-time psychiatrist expert at family therapy, three mental health assistants, and a specialist in human relations who had extensive experience in community organization work. Subsequently, we added a specialist in group work and acquired the part-time services of a specialist in counseling who was also interested in school consultation and education programs.

The range of talents and interests was a manifestation of our fundamental belief that many types of knowledge and skills are needed to develop programs for children. Each professional chosen was a specialist in a field and committed not only to exercising or practicing a specialty but also to teaching and sharing his or her expertise with others less trained and experienced. We stressed this teaching and training function as a primary responsibility and commitment of each staff member. Every specialist had responsibility to teach and develop skills of the generalists, primary therapists, and primary caretakers with whom they worked, whether these were other staff members of the mental health center or staff of other agencies. All the professionals discovered that the area of common skills and activities was much greater than the training of the various traditional disciplines had acknowledged.

As an instance, take the word "therapy." Psychiatrists do it. Psychologists do it, but supposedly of a less intense variety. Social workers do "casework" or use the "helping process." Guidance and vocational counselors "counsel," as do clergymen. Now there are differences in the meaning of these words, and they do connote differences in methods, focus, and technique. In fact, however, the behaviors of mental health workers with clients are most influenced by experience, the mode or fashion of the particular clinical setting, and the individual style of the worker.

Role diffusion, "how come I'm doing all these different kinds of things I didn't think I was trained or expected to do?" and role overlap, "how come she's doing something I thought I had the exclusive training or right to do?" will occur and must be dealt with repeatedly. Anxiety develops because of ambiguity around role definition, territorial encroachment, and competition which involves not only the relationship between paraprofessionals and professionals but among professional disciplines, as well.

How did we deal with these problems? The administrator in such a situation has several functions to perform. He has to preach and practice the beliefs and values he holds. If he believes in no jargon, then he must be sure to talk straight. If he believes that many people have skills to be helpful with children and families, then he must really support the fact that others can treat and care for families and children.

The director of the Children and Family Unit had decided to expend his efforts in three major ways. First and foremost, he was personally available to the staff for discussion and support, particularly about issues about role: diffusion, overlap, uncertainty. Second, he made himself responsible for socializing the unit to values and beliefs that the service professed. When an administrator includes other staff members in decision and policy making, it will facilitate socialization and promote cohesiveness among members. Making policy is literally a concrete expression of a belief or value in terms that are oriented toward action. If the group that is to be involved in carrying out much action can also be involved in the policy making, then the policy becomes an expression of a jointly held value. This policy has a greater likelihood of not only being carried out but also of binding members of a group to it and through it to each other.

A third way in which the director expended his administrative energies was in helping persons find specific goal-directed tasks that were congruent with the practical blend of two ingredients: (1) policies and responsibilities of the unit and (2) interests, skills, and competence of the person. In the best of instances, what results is that people's activities are related to what needs to be done, what the value system says should be done, what the practical realities of time, people, money, and space dictate can be done, and what people like to do and are good at. Losing the comfort of the well-defined uniform of the old role is made somewhat easier by the trade-off for the custom-tailored uniform of a new role.

PROBLEMS IN IMPLEMENTATION: ADMINISTRATIVE
AND PRACTICAL

What sort of problems did we encounter in forming such a unit and in attempting to carry out its goals? We divide these into problems that occurred within the structure and context of the mental health center and problems related to outside influences. The latter refer to such matters as the influence of the county and state mental health regulations, the federal regulations and guidelines, the availability of adequate funds, and the availability of qualified personnel.

One major initial and continuing problem centered around our existence as a maverick service unit. In accordance with the NIMH guidelines, our mental health center had five essential services and several optional services. These guidelines, however, do not specify a separate children's service. Therefore, we were repeatedly faced with problems of our administrative identity in terms of other service units within the center as well as outside agencies and clients. We have already described our reasons for organizing the Children and Family Unit as a separate entity. Those reasons remained valid throughout the first 5 years of the center's existence which are covered in this report. The validity of reasons did not magically avoid obstacles in terms of acceptance, recognition of this type of organizational structure, nor did sound reasoning obviate difficulties in carrying out the mission and goals of the unit. Within the center, the Children and Family Unit had administrative and service parity and the relationships among other service directors and line staff were good. We emphasized that our staff be available to the staff of other units to respond to the problems encountered in the evaluation and care of children and families. That we were easy to get to and available to help was one of the primary ways we communicated our role. Face-to-face availability was one of the means we used to try to diminish the resistance and resentment that some staff had about the unit's primary responsibility being a consultative one rather than a direct service unit for all children.

Because we were a maverick service, we encountered significant difficulties in relation to the local, state, and federal administrative bodies. Mental health centers are required to submit official reports to county and state offices describing the various functions and services and proposing budget estimates for future support of services. In these reports, the Children and Family Unit did not exist as a distinct budgetary entity. This is because the system as established would not allow it and would not recognize it. There was no way that the Children and Family Unit could be reported as a separate autonomous unit in the center with its own personnel and budget. Budgetary allocations had to be distributed according to the five essential services described by the mental health center act.

Record keeping was another problem. We were faced with the question of how we could obtain adequate information about children and families who applied for service and what happened from the time of initial contact until they were terminated or lost to follow-up. This problem was shared by the whole center and the record-keeping system went through a number of changes until it reached its final state. It took several years for an effective, adequate record system to be developed.

One of our initial tasks in the role of advocacy for children within the center was to work with the staff of the research and evaluation unit to modify the initial patient record form so that it would be usable for children. One of our staff members, a research assistant, worked with the directors of both units to develop a data form which would adequately and accurately record information in those instances in which children appear as the primary client. This new form included information which had previously not been obtained: identification of the child as the patient, the child's school and grade, his special class status if applicable, whether the child was living with the natural or foster parents, and the name and relationship of the informant. These and other significant data were incorporated into the initial intake form and accomplished the first step in adequately accounting for children who applied for service.

However, this did not provide complete knowledge of how many children and families were initially applying for service, how many received what kind of service, who failed to keep initial or subsequent appointments, and so forth. As part of our responsibility, the staff of the Children and Family Unit decided we needed more information than the basic demographic data recorded at intake. We needed more immediate clinical data as clients applied to know what was happening to them. As described above, our stance was that of responding to requests from the primary therapist for help about this or that child or family.

Since we did not provide a large amount of direct service in the early years, the staff of our unit did not know all the children who were being serviced by the mental health center. There were occasions when we were not consulted by the primary therapist either because he felt no need to do so or because the child and family dropped out of service after only a brief engagement. At other times, after consulting us, the primary therapist might be unable to follow-up and work with the child or family or they refused to be involved in further service. At other times, we misjudged the capacity of the primary therapist to deal with the child and family that presented difficult problems or we misjudged the seriousness of the problem that the child and family presented and expected too much of the primary therapist. When we were able to identify such a situation, we could take over the management of the case. However, when such cases were not identified, we were not able to do anything about them. Because we lacked a good method of being informed about the total population applying for service and their careers in the center, a number of children and their families were lost.

The practical problem can be stated as follows. Since our unit was not a first line unit at the point of application and entry, and since we only saw those children and families whom our staff asked us to see, how could we know about the children who apply whom we are never asked about? These could be children and families who apply and never show, who apply and show but drop out, who apply and are serviced and terminated. They can be the most successful, the never engaged, or the worst failures that others are afraid of or ashamed to ask for help with. There are a variety of approaches to solving this problem, several of which we tried over the years. These can be classified into indirect and direct methods.

INDIRECT METHOD

One of the first indirect solutions alluded to above was the general and special record system. In such a system, all client applicants are recorded and their status is monitored in an ongoing way. In addition to our work around a general record system which was never totally effective for that task, we developed a special record system that our unit kept on children and families. We included certain basic data for all children and families who applied and were in the process of developing a particular system to follow-up and record the client's career in the center. Such a system included both children about who we consulted as well as those we did not. In addition to the initial intake form, special supplementary information developed particularly for the Children and Family Unit record system was collected from all children at the point of entry.

DIRECT METHODS

Direct methods use various approaches based on some direct personal contact of one group of staff with another, or with the clients themselves. One approach was to attach the liaison person from the Children and Family Unit to one or more of the several functioning teams of the psychosocial clinic. A member of our unit would meet regularly with members of the psychosocial clinic team at one of their scheduled meetings. The purpose of such meetings was to review cases of children and families, answer questions concerning diagnosis and management, arrange future consultation interviews to be carried out by one of the Children and Family Unit staff. This approach was helpful but there still remained the significant number of children about whom we were uninformed.

The second direct approach involved the establishment of an evaluation team of child specialists who would see all child and family applicants at the point of intake, and then make a decision of a triage nature as to whether or not these children and families would be referred to the generalist in the psychosocial clinic or to be directly cared for by the staff of the Children and Family Unit. This method was implemented for a brief period of time but was not given an adequate trial. It still seems to be a useful approach to acquire direct knowledge of the applicant population as well as a parsimonious way of deploying scarce manpower.

THE COMBINED APPROACH

As our unit took on greater direct responsibility for providing service to families of mentally retarded children in the catchment area, we evolved a more satisfactory records procedure. Our unit assumed the initial direct responsibility for the retarded child and his family. In order to have adequate and complete records of these clients, we developed an approach which we subsequently extended to all children whether with mental health or with mental retardation difficulties.

The first step occurred at the point of entry to the center. A copy of every child's intake application was sent to our unit from whatever unit the child and family had first applied for service. Thus, whether the entry point was the crisis center, psychosocial clinic, or in fewer instances, the partial hospitalization program, a copy of the initial intake form was sent to the Children and Family Unit intake worker. A weekly screening and review session was held by the senior staff of the Children and Family Unit. The administrative assistant of the unit had responsibility for the actual mechanics of record keeping and monitoring of decisions arising from the review session. In addition, we strongly encouraged the presence and participation of the staff of those units who had the initial responsibility for the children whose applications we were to review. The sessions consisted of a paper review of the initial applications for service. This application included a statement of the patient's presenting problem, recent history, and brief statements of the functioning of the child socially, in school, and in the family. Some data concerning the family, both demographically and functionally, was often obtained. If the staff of the initiating unit was present at our screening session, we encouraged their opinions and participation in arriving at one of several decisions:

1. Return the application, recommending that the child and family receive the initial and ongoing service from the unit of origin.
2. Return the application, recommending that after the original service unit does the initial evaluation, a member of our unit be involved in a consultative and planning interview. Decision for continuing service would derive from that session.
3. Recommend the complete transfer of responsibility for the child and

family to the Children and Family Unit for evaluation and continuing service.

4. Recommend that the original unit with or without assistance from a member of the Children and Family Unit make referral of the family to another agency which we judged could provide service more appropriate to this family's needs.

5. Ask members of the initial service unit to meet and discuss the client's application to clear up questions or confusions before arriving at any further recommendations of types 1 to 4 above.

MENTAL RETARDATION PROGRAM

In 1969, the Pennsylvania State regulations required that mental health centers provide comprehensive services to mentally retarded children whose presenting problems were primarily emotional or mental in nature. However, grant requirements stipulated that there be a designated mental retardation service and mental retardation staff. This is in line with the same principle we applied to children, in general, that in the past retarded children have received little or no service and to ensure that such service was provided, a designated administrative unit and staff responsible for carrying out service to the retarded children was necessary. We satisfied the grant requirements and accomplished integration of our overall approach by including a mental retardation staff within the Children and Family Unit. The total program was the responsibility of the original director of the Children and Family Unit. There was, however, a specific staff hired in designated positions to be the primary service givers to retarded children and their families. We maintained the belief, in principle and practice, of the one door of entry. Further, we did not want to separate our staff totally; to have one group of staff only seeing mentally disturbed children and another group of staff seeing exclusively mentally retarded children and their families. The risk for emotional disturbance is even higher among retarded children than nonretarded. Therefore, we insisted that our total staff make every possible effort to provide the integrated services to both kinds of clients, whatever their primary presenting problem. We applied our principle of using paraprofessionals, by hiring staff who had been trained in child care training programs and who had previous experience at St. Christopher's Hospital in working in the home with families of retarded and handicapped children. These staff were called *family counselors* for administrative purposes but carried out many of the same functions as our mental health assistants.

Families with mentally retarded children present special problems if the children are in the moderate or severely retarded range. We needed to ensure that these children received adequate physical and neurological evaluations. We accomplished this by a contractual arrangement with the Handicapped Children's Unit of St. Christopher's Hospital for Children which is the pediatric hospital of Temple University. Since the Handicapped Children's Unit had been established and served as a regional center for several states, it was logical to use these existing diagnostic services for those handicapped children who were applicants to our center. This unit had a full range of skilled personnel including child neurologists, pediatricians specializing in habilitation medicine, social workers, and psychologists, audiologists, speech therapists, and physiotherapists. It would have been foolhardy and impossible for us to try to recruit personnel of the quality and skill needed to provide these comparable services.

In maximizing the effect of our staff, we emphasized such issues as the provision of home service and the establishment of institutional linkages for the families so they might develop connections with special education or rehabilitation centers. In work with families of retarded children, there is often in addition to therapeutic function, a significant case planning and management function. Paraprofessional workers, under the supervision of an experienced social worker in the area of mental retardation helped the family make plans and take steps to get connected with those community agencies and services, scarce as they are, which would be appropriate for their mentally retarded child.

Further, we found that many children referred for mental health problems from schools had low IQ scores and hence were labeled mentally retarded and put in special classes for the retarded educable. This represents yet another example of social extrusion. (See discussion in Chapter 12.) We felt it was our responsibility not only to deal with the clinical issue in terms of direct service for these children but also to get at some of the system issues within the school, in other words, the whole notion of the RE class. In many cases, this class serves as a wastebasket or dumping ground for low status children, children who have a variety of problems and who, in addition, score low on an IQ test. This score justifies the administrative decision to place them in a special class. Our major role in our consultative and intervention function in the school was to attempt to provide advocacy for these children so that wherever possible they could be moved into a regular class if we could demonstrate that they could manage the work and if the school was able to provide extra support and help. (See Chapter 6 for a discussion of center educational services.)

REFERENCES

1. Glaser FB: Our place: design for a day program. Am J Orthopsychiatry 39:827–841, 1969
2. Panzetta, AF: Community Mental Health: Myth and Reality. Philadelphia, Lea & Febiger, 1970
3. Lynch M, Gardner EA, Felzer SB: The role of indigenous personnel as clinic therapists: training and implication for new careers. Arch Gen Psychiatry 19:428–434, 1968
4. United States Congress: Public Law 88–164: Mental Retardation Facilities and Community Mental Health Center Construction Act of 1963. Washington, D.C. Govt. Printing Office, 1964
5. Report of the Joint Commission on Mental Health of Children. Crisis in child mental health: challenge for the 1970's. New York, Harper & Row, 1969
6. Rosenblum G: Can children's services flourish in a comprehensive community mental health center? J Am Acad Child Psychiatry 8:485–492, 1969
7. Group for the Advancement of Psychiatry. Crisis in child mental health: a critical assessment. New York, GAP Publication No. 82, 1972, p 111
8. Glasscote R, Fishman M, Sonis M: Children and Mental Health Centers: Programs, Problems, Prospects. Washington, D.C. Joint Information Service of American Psychiatric Association, and National Association for Mental Health, 1972
9. McDermott JF, Harrison SI, Schrager J, Wilson PT: Social class and mental illness in children: observations of blue collar families. Am J Orthopsychiatry 35:500–508, 1965
10. Harrison SI, McDermott, JF, Wilson PT, Schrager J: Social class and mental illness in children: choice of treatment. Arch Gen Psychiatry 13:411–417, 1965
11. Adams P, McDonald N: Clinical cooling out of poor people. Am J Orthopsychiatry 38:457–463, 1968
12. Satir VM: Conjoint Family Therapy: A Guide to Theory and Technique. Palo Alto, Science and Behavior Books, 1964
13. Minuchin S, Montalvo B, Guerney BG Jr, Rosman BL, Shumer F: Families of the Slums. New York, Basic Books, 1967
14. Haley J: Family therapy. Int J Psychiatry 9:233–242, 1970
15. Albee G: The relation of conceptual models to manpower needs. In Cowen AL, Gardner EA, Zax M (eds): Emergent Approaches to Mental Health Problems. New York, Appleton, 1967, p 63–73
16. Rae-Grant Q, Gladwin T, Bowers E: Mental health, social competence and the war on poverty. Am J Orthopsychiatry 36:652–664, 1966

Part II

Consultation

4

Mental Health Intervention in the Schools: Some Conceptual Options

Mental health intervention in the schools can be based on a number of conceptual options. We have chosen to examine five: the educational option, the handicapped option, the illness-treatment option, the socialization option, and the system option. These options are typically used, though not explicitly stated, when schools and consultants view the mental health of pupils. Each option carries with it its own particular operations and results.

At the outset, mental health workers and educators are faced with a communication problem. This problem arises from assumptions and habits of thought, as well as from differences in daily tasks. One analogy of this issue is the difficulty two apparently similar groups of people have in communicating when they speak different dialects of the same language. An inherent mutual responsibility of both educators and mental health consultants is to reiterate the invaluable semantic question: "What do you mean by that?" The first and continuing problem of any dialogue is *not* defining the problem. Rather it is agreeing on a language by which problems can be defined and through which all other meaningful communication may take place.

THE EDUCATIONAL OPTION

This is obviously the most usual option adopted by educators because it is "natural" to their state. Hence, they automatically invoke it even when they confront issues that are relatively foreign to their background and experience, such as emotional or behavioral problems. From this vantage point, children are to be moved from a state of ignorance to a state of knowledge. The procedures used involve that which is broadly termed *education*. These are carried out by action of the teacher and administrator. The means used are the curriculum, which is mainly general, explicit, and formal, and control procedures, which tend to be individualized, implicit, and less formalized. The outcome of these actions, individually and collectively, is to produce result criteria which dichotimize children into successes and failures (this can sometimes be construed to mean "good" or "bad" children).

Under this option, behavior problems tend to be of two sorts. One type is disturbed, emotionally upset, and "sick" behavior. This behavior falls within the province of the counselor and the psychological or special services. The second type is "bad" behavior, which usually tends to be antiauthoritarian, aggressive, truant, and possibly destructive. Initially, the teacher is responsible for "correcting" this behavior, but ultimately it becomes the province of the disciplinarian, attendance officer, and enforcement personnel, sometimes involving the police and court. Often there is a crossing over from one viewpoint to another, both regarding the same behavior in different children or different behavior in the same child. Glasser has provided an analysis of the school that is similar in some respects.[1]

This option is highly rational in its approach. Feelings and their effects on both behavior and learning are underemphasized, whereas knowledge of subject matter or right or wrong behavior is stressed. There is also great emphasis placed on altering the logistics of the system by the manipulation of school environment through schedule changes, classroom cycling, homogeneous or heterogeneous groupings, open classrooms, individualized instruction, employment of new hardware, and programmed methods. (More recently, certain creative approaches have been developed in remedying the neglected feelings through the development of affective curriculum projects.)[2]

Remedies that tend to proceed from the educational option are of an incremental or additional type. Those applying the remedy seem to be saying, "If we could only add knowledge, understanding, control, motivation, parental concern, then the behavior would change or the learning would increase, or both would occur." More desperate remedies tend to take the form of admonitions, penalties, threats, suspensions, and other punishment directed at the child or his parents, or both.

THE HANDICAPPED OPTION

The handicapped option is an important, sophisticated, and refined subform of the educational option. The handicapped viewpoint is used within the framework of special education, which is a rubric given to remedial intervention directed toward handicapped children. Reger et al[3] indicate two connotations of the notion of handicapped: an absolute one and a relative one. The latter notion is related to the social context of the time and place, which determines whether or not a condition is handicapping. Reger cogently argues that schools and teachers should exert the responsibility they have for defining handicap, and planning intervention in educationally meaningful terms. Although his intervention strategies focus on learning problems especially as they relate to language, nevertheless the operational terms Reger use are highly neurophysiologically oriented. He stresses the need to evaluate and remedy handicaps in the area of visual, sensory-motor, auditory, and associational processes.

Like the more general educational option, in which ignorance and bad behavior are the child's possessions and belong to him, so in this more sophisticated option, the handicap is still the child's own but at a more molecular, anatomic, and physiological level. The issue of whether the child possesses or is possessed by the handicap is one that is decided by the particular bias of the individual evaluator or teacher. Handicap thus belongs to the child, though not necessarily brought on by him. The handicap operates to some degree beyond his control, and with more subtle and complicated handicaps, beyond his specific awareness of their operation. He is only aware of his inability to read, or to discriminate auditory tones, or to pay attention. In this view, the handicap is not resolved spontaneously and does not respond to the conscious solo efforts of the child's will.

The result of this option is a strong emphasis on the evaluation of perceptual and motor behavior, both simple and complex. Careful attention is provided to the physical structure of the classroom, and even more to the structure of curriculum material and content. These tools and techniques generally imply one or both of the following strategies: (1) to overcome the handicap, strengthening the weakness or (2) compensatory emphasis on assets, strengthening the strengths.

In the area of emotions and behavior, this option is strongly influenced by learning theory and behavioral techniques. Emphasis is placed on classroom structuring and clearly defined rules, consistently applied by the teacher. Operationalizing the maxim "behavior has consequences" is pursued with vigor. By contrast, there is much less emphasis on the interpersonal aspects of the teacher-child relationship and on the whole affective dimension. Even more than in the educational option, in the handicapped one advances a more sophisticated and scientifically supported rationalism.

THE ILLNESS-TREATMENT OPTION

This is probably the most frequently invoked option when mental health or psychiatric consultants confront a problem.[4,5] This choice is a logical one, since by training and experience, psychiatrists tend to see themselves as healers of "sickness." Further, psychodynamic theories are dominant in psychiatry and psychology, both in terms of the explanation of personality and as a theory of therapy. Alternative terms to sickness are "emotional disturbance" and "behavior disorder." Both of these terms are usually related to a psychopathology model, which is basically medical.

Though less than in the educational option, children are once again objects toward which action is directed, usually from the consultant by means of the teacher, counselor, or principal. This conceptualization tends to dichotimize children as the educational option did. Here, however, the division is into well-sick, with a strong emphasis on the sick and pathologic. For the educator, this well-sick dichotomy is more likely to really mean bad-good, than the dichotomy of success-failure did in the educational framework.

The illness-treatment option in the main locates problems "inside the skin" of the child. The individual child is emphasized somewhat isolated from his social context or is viewed in a limited two-person relationship such as his relationship with his teacher, with his parent, or peers.

This option also affects the relationship between the mental health consultant and the school counselor, psychologist, social worker, or other personnel. It is in the domain of these special service personnel that the sick or disturbed child finally falls. Alliances of an overt or covert nature often occur between the consultant and these personnel. Since they, in turn, often have a safety valve and referral function for the school, they may push the consultant into a direct treatment role as a means of relieving the pressure on them. Furthermore, special service personnel usually occupy a sideline position relative to the decision-making processes of the school. If the consultant's alliance with them is too close, he may also lessen his accessibility to teachers and administrators.

Remedies that are applied by this option are directed to changing something inside the child—feelings and attitudes. If the remedy is wrongly applied to the teacher as well, it frequently involves adding an additional role by making her a "therapist." The consultant using this option needs to avoid the hazard of misapplying what is relevant in a one-to-one clinical therapeutic activity to the setting of a classroom in which one teacher and many children are gathered together for educational, and not treatment purposes.

Another possible result of those remedies issuing from the therapeutic option which focuses on the teacher more than on the children is to "sensitize" the teacher to signs of disturbance and to "persuade" her that what she called "bad" or "lazy" behavior is really "illness," or the results of an emotional disturbance over which the child has diminished control. Although this may increase the teacher's understanding, it may also make her feel more helpless when faced with such behavior and in that sense promotes no one's mental health—child or teacher. Unfortunately, the most abused outcome of this option allows the school's staff to label a child "sick" or "disturbed." This turns him into a legitimate candidate for referral to a clinic or therapist who treats sick or disturbed children.

THE SOCIALIZATION OPTION

Socialization includes all the knowledge, skills, and abilities transmitted by precept and example, formally and informally, consciously and unconsciously, to the end of accomplishing an adaptive "fit" between the person and his social environment. This social environment is construed in successively more global terms with each stage of development. Competence as a positive adaptive concept in the general sense was introduced by White.[6] Clausen[7] edited a recent work in which social competence is viewed from several perspectives by various writers.

The socialization option derives from academic and experimental psychology, general learning and social learning theory, developmental theory and sociology. It is in contrast to the aforementioned options which had strongly educational or medical origins. Recently, concepts of operant conditioning have come to play an important role in this option, and there is much in the socialization concept that can be construed in behavioral terms. Basically, however, the socialization option is broader and more general and hence subsumes much of what is contained in a behavioral option. By no means does this mean that both options have identical assumptions or theoretical constructs. The socialization option includes a consideration of the whole spectrum of behavior rather than focusing on just one special aspect. This orientation is less likely to lead to dichotomous thinking, since the emphasis is on positive factors, that is, competence, rather than negative ones. Even more important, this orientation takes into account the social context rather than highlighting the symptoms of a person, or whether he achieves or fails to obtain certain grades as evidence of success or failure.

The interaction between the person and the group or among group members is central to this position, as is the person's adaptation to the school as a social institution. Roles, expectations, peer influences, positive and negative sanctions, and modeling behavior are relevant concepts within this option. The contingency paradigm "If this . . . than that." becomes crucial in analyzing what is wrong with the situation as well as in planning solutions. We may examine this concept of socialization concretely with a simple nontrivial example. When a 5- or 6-year-old child enters school, it is assumed, incorrectly for certain children, that he will have achieved through his previous socializing experiences a capacity to *sit still* for some fairly protracted period of time. It is further assumed that he has achieved some ability in listening and in discriminating between two types of communication and in responding appropriately to each. One type of communication is *directional:* "Do this"; "don't do that"; "pick up your blue crayon." The second type of communication is *informational:* "All Gaul is divided into three parts." "Blue, red, and yellow are primary colors."

Proper and adequate response to each type of communication brings particular types of rewards. Proper response to directional communication is rewarded by all the factors: praise, high conduct marks, position of privilege vis-à-vis teachers or peers, pride of family, connoted by the phrase, "good boy." Proper response to informational types of communication, including remembering, recall correctly on demand, integrating, satisfying innate curiosity, developing cognitive mastery, is rewarded by all the nuances connoted by the phrase "smart boy."

However, some children do not come to school equipped with these skills in any immediate and functional form. Usually the social program of the school or society is not formulated taking them into account. They become, therefore, socially maladapted to school. Secondarily, the child's behavior and too often the child himself is considered a nuisance. The teacher becomes frustrated and the child reaps the dubious rewards of disapproval by teachers and parents. Such children experience dejection and rejection, react with defiance or withdrawal, and then truly become emotionally maladapted.

Remedies suggested by this type of orientation are not primarily directed at enhancing the child's content learning as are the remedies of the educational model. Neither are remedies directed primarily at changes of pathologic, sick, or disturbed behavior by internal affective and motivational change as in the pathologic-therapeutic model. From this orientation, remedies are aimed at enhancing the child's ability to perceive, understand, and execute the roles of the "school game" and become an effective "player." The focus is on enabling the child to learn how to learn, or to learn how to behave, or both. Helping children to learn the rules or to "make it," however, still emphasizes that onus for change is on the child, and he must meet the criteria of the system. In general, in this as in the previous options, those criteria and assumptions remain unexamined. The major stress is placed on the manipulation of environmental contingencies, especially the social ones that affect or alter the child's behavior. There is also explicit conscious use of the modeling powers of other persons, both adults and children.

At this point, we should note that the first four options preserve the established attitude that maintains psychologic distance between the interveners, that is, school personnel, consultants, and parents, and the objects of the interventions—the children. To a greater or lesser degree, this we-they distance is emphasized and often highly valued. The result of this stance is arbitrarily and artificially to exclude the adults and their behaviors from the psychosocial field, much as the laboratory experimenter chooses to isolate some variables for purposes of simplification and manageability. Essentially, this exclusion is merely a subjective option in the mind of the excluders—the adults. In reality, these excluded adults are an integral part of the factors affecting the children, whether or not they explicitly advert to them.

THE SYSTEM OPTION

A system is defined as a set of connected or interdependent things which form a complex unity and are arranged according to some plan. The use of the word "system" here should be distinguished from its application in general systems theory which has been developed and used over the last decade. This latter theory was expounded in one of its earliest forms by the biologist, von Bertalanffy[8] and has been applied in economics, in business management, to strategies of the Cold War, and more recently, to the behavioral sciences. General systems theory has attempted to develop constructs and properties to apply to all systems. The specific conceptual tool has been to detail the analogies common to all systems, horizontally across disciplines of knowledge and vertically from the microsystem to the macrosystem. Important terms used in general systems theory include *input, information processing, feedback, storage,* and *message processes.*

To emphasize the system changes the focus of conceptualization. Each of the four previous conceptual options could be typified as a particular system, for example, the educational "system," but the emphasis in each of those options was of the *adjectival term* or the modifier rather than on the "system as system." This conceptual option proposes to view the school and school mental health intervention not by emphasizing school (the educational aspect) nor mental health (treatment-illness) but by highlighting the notion of *system*. The result of such a view is to raise to the level of relevance such questions as the following:

What do we mean by system? What are the characteristics of the system? What are the values and goals of the system? What are the methods of achieving these goals and values? What are the components of the system? What are the processes of the system? What are the roles of importance in the system, formal and informal, major and subordinate? What are the rules, explicit and implicit? What are the decision-making processes? What are the communications processes? How do they work?

In this option, the central question is "How does the relative perspective of each of us who are members of, or who look at and speak about the system, determine what we see and say?" In turn, how are our own attitudes and behaviors determined by our roles in the system?

By explicitly dealing with system as they key concept, it is no longer possible to adopt the psychological luxury of distancing ourselves from "the others" in the system. The essential point here is the notion of mutual influence through interaction. The basic law of system can be stated as follows: *everybody is in on everything.* Reciprocal relationships are central events in the reality of any system and are necessary resultants of adopting this conceptual option. Each member and group in a system is influenced by and influences the other. Teachers not only "do to" children, children "do to" teachers. It is this interaction, this "way of doing business together" that constitutes the system in operation at one level. The same approach may be applied to faculty-principal interaction. The diagram in Figure 4.1 illustrates a series of systematic interactions.

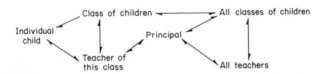

Fig. 4.1.   The arrows in the diagram are bidirectional and involve persons and both small and large groups. One could complicate and more faithfully replicate the reality by adding transactional arrows between a child and counselor, between curriculum specialist and teacher, between child and a class or child and principal, between principal and superintendent, between parent and teacher or parent and child, between principal and community groups, etc.

This option leads to the reformulation and relabeling of various aspects of the school. One can now use the terms *components* and *processes* for describing the school. Argyris[9] calls the steady state properties of an organizational structure (components) the "what" and the dynamic properties (processes) the "how" of organizations. Components can be both human—children, teachers, principals, parents and non-human—curriculum, schedules, and rooms. Emphasizing components makes any intervention more specific and tangible (e.g., a program directed toward all kindergarten children and teachers or aimed at a revision of the social studies curriculum to include the human motivation for behavior.)

Processes are less tangible and more pervasive than components. They cut vertically and horizontally through a school and can involve all components. Processes are more likely to involve interactions between components and are labeled so as to characterize the nature of the interaction, for example, communication, or to highlight the nature of the relationships between components, for example, positive-alliance, conflict, superior-subordinate. Status relationships, role expectancies and behaviors, and rules are the vehicles through which the various processes are expressed and made concrete. Interventions directed at identifying and analyzing processes lead to increased understanding of the school's social organization, the decision-making process, and the reward and sanction system. This can result in a more rational and conscious use of current processes, or appropriate changes and modifications.[10] A focus on the system, its components, and processes brings hazards as well: a tendency toward diffuseness and vagueness, and a marked increase in anxiety and protective behavior. Often there is a lack of tangible results because there has not been a clear specification of what changes are being sought and how these changes are to be effected. To use this approach as a basis for intervention requires considerable knowledge, persistence, and skill on the part of consultant and school staff.

REFERENCES

1. Glasser W: Schools Without Failure. New York, Harper & Row, 1969
2. Newberg NA: Impact of affective education on Philadelphia schools. Educ Opp Forum 1:17–37, 1969
3. Reger R, Schroeder W, Uschold C: Special Education: Children with Learning Problems. New York, Oxford Univ. Press, 1968
4. Berlin I: Mental health consultation in the schools: who can do it and why. Community Ment Health J 1:19–22, 1965

5. Newman RG: Psychological Consultation in the Schools. New York, Basic Books, 1967
6. White RW: Motivation reconsidered: the concept of competence. Psychol Rev 66:297–333, 1959
7. Clausen JA, (ed): Socialization and Society. Boston, Little, Brown, 1968
8. von Bertalanffy L: General Systems Theory. New York, Braziller, 1968
9. Argyris C: On the effectiveness of research and development organization. Am Sci 56:344–355, 1968
10. Schein EH: Process Consultation: Its Role in Organization Development. Reading, Mass., Addison-Wesley, 1969

5

Problems and Processes of
School Consultation

Imagine, if you will, the following all too familiar set of circumstances. The principal of a local public school in your community calls up the clinic where you work and says that he has become very interested in developing a collaborative program involving mental health personnel in his school. You and some of your staff, eager to get out of the press of seeing all of those difficult patients in the clinic, respond enthusiastically to this initial contact. You also begin to feel, perhaps somewhat smugly, that at least some of the people "out there" like your principal have begun to get the "message." The message is that mental health is everybody's business and that schools are a very logical place for mental health interventions. You probably have met this particular principal before at various meetings around town, and you may even have discussed the case of an individual child or two with him. Now he seems to want something more than that and you begin to view him as a potential, if not actual, convert to your way of thinking. Your way of thinking generally means some kind of primary preventive approach that deals with larger numbers of children than can effectively be handled in a child guidance clinic. A meeting is arranged and a process has begun which leads to the development of another school consultation program.

A condensed version of this paper was published in the Journal of the American Academy of Child Psychiatry, 11 (4): 694–704, 1972. We wish to acknowledge the contribution of Anne Glass, A.C.S.W. to the section of this chapter dealing with School Discipline Teams.

In this chapter, we would like to share with you the impressions of two child psychiatrists who are battle-weary veterans of more than a dozen school consultation programs. We do not propose to be exhaustive or to present the "last word" about school consultation. We admit to being biased, perhaps even cynical, and certainly not rigorously "scientific" in our presentation. Rather, our approach is impressionistic, intuitive, anecdotal, and experiential. Our experience as school consultants has been exclusively in urban schools, and primarily in schools in low socioeconomic neighborhoods. Some of our colleagues who work in suburban or semirural school systems suggest that there may be fewer problems in those settings, or that at least the problems appear to be more manageable.

In order to illustrate the early discussions and negotiations which lead to the implementation of a school consultation program, we re-create the peregrinations of a fictitious, but typical consultant, Dr. C. We begin with the initial telephone contact, and then continue through a condensed version of subsequent phases which characterize the beginnings of a program.

INITIAL CONTACT

Mr. J.:   Hello, Dr. C., I'm Mr. J., principal of the XYZ School. I've been trying to reach you for a few days. I've been referred to you by Mr. H. of the school board who tells me that you're interested in getting involved in some school programs. I'd like to talk over some ideas with you.

Dr. C.:   Yes, I'm sorry you had a hard time getting in touch with me. That's because I've been spending so much time away from my office and in the schools. (This is a variant of an ancient law of physics too often forgotten by consultants: No one can be in two places at the same time, or, be very careful about how many commitments you take on.) What did you have in mind?

Mr. J.:   Well, we have a number of problem children here, and we'd like some kind of help with them. We could send them to your clinic, but it takes a long time to get them in. We thought maybe you could work with them here.

Dr. C.:   I see. Work with them in what way?

Mr. J.:   Maybe in some kind of group. We don't have any money to set up a special class for them, but we could bring them together once or twice a week in group meetings.

Dr. C.:   Well, let's arrange an appointment to talk about it. Suppose I come over there. Is next Tuesday at 2:00 PM all right?

Mr. J.:   Yes, that's fine. We'll see you then.

Dr. C. arrives at the XYZ School, an elementary grade school 1 mile from his clinic. The children are just coming in from recess with much pushing, shoving, and noise. The teachers are vainly struggling to keep them in orderly lines. The school is about 70 years old, generally shabby, with some broken windows, and standard graffiti in evidence. Dr. C. goes to the principal's office and introduces himself.

Secretary: Yes, could you wait a few minutes? Mr. J. had to take yard duty, today. Three of our teachers are out sick. (Schools and consultants often operate on different time schedules. A consultant who is a psychiatrist, particularly views time within the context of a 50-minute hour, interprets lateness as resistance, and must have a certain order in his practice. Time is less well protected for principals; intrusions are frequent, and emergencies are almost constant. The best results in a consultation program may occur when each party handles his time more like the other.)

As he waits, Dr. C. looks at the faculty bulletin board, which among other things notes "Faculty Meeting on Friday, February 23rd (already passed) will include visit from Research Department of the School District to discuss Iowa Test Scores. On March 23rd, a distinguished guest speaker will speak on the Problems of a Disadvantaged Child." Mr. J. arrives. After some introductory and courtesy remarks, Mr. J. goes on.

Mr. J.:   We have a big problem here, kids are disrupting classes, running around, not sitting still, not learning well. We try to get them to behave, but nothing seems to work.

Dr. C.:   What have you tried?

Mr. J.:   The usual things. They are sent to my office. I reprimand them, and occasionally I suspend a child and get the parent in. I talk to the parents about their child's behavior, but they don't seem to care much. And even if they do care, it's also hard for them to come in because they work. Some of the children don't have fathers, and there just doesn't seem to be any discipline in the home. I'm sure you've heard all of this before. (The consultant probably has, but it's important to listen, not only to promote rapport, but also because the principal's theories about children and their families determine his actions toward them. His behavior often sets the tone for the school.)

Dr. C. at this point asks questions about the size of the school, faculty-student ratio, counseling services in the school, and the availability of psychological testing. He essentially learns that there are inadequate resources in all of these dimensions.

Dr. C.:   Getting back to your original question, how many children are you most concerned about, and what grades are they in?

Mr. J.:   Sometimes, I think I could send you all of them, but right now we seem to have about 10 or 12 fifth and sixth graders who are giving us the most trouble. Some of them are in my office every day. The other day one of them pulled the fire alarm. He's suspended now. We have a total of 6 fifth and sixth grade classes, so we're talking about an average of two children per class who are the biggest problem.

Dr. C.: Does anything in particular, other than their behavior, distinguish these children from the others?

Mr. J.: Well, they're all boys, they seem to come from the least interested families, and they are poor students.

Dr. C.: Of your fifth and sixth grade teachers, are there any of them who send their children to you more frequently than others?

Mr. J.: Well, perhaps Miss Taylor does. She's new, just out of school. Well meaning, but kind of naïve. Of course, we have a turnover rate of about 40 percent per year in our teachers, so it's not all that unusual to be new. (Here the consultant might have inquired about the absentee rate among teachers, which in some schools is higher than that of the pupils.)

(The telephone rings. The secretary buzzes the principal, and there is a brief interruption while he discusses some problem in the school's lunch program with the caller.)

Dr. C.: I noted something on the bulletin board about a discussion on the disadvantaged child. Does that kind of thing prove valuable?

Mr. J.: We try to have some staff development here, usually by discussing interesting topics at faculty meetings. We have no money to do anything beyond that. The last talk from the District Testing Office didn't go over too well. The teachers seem to feel that the School District spends too much money on research and doing standardized testing, not enough on actually doing something about reading. (Messages coming from District Headquarters or "Downtown" are likely to receive a lukewarm reception, at best, in the local schools. The bearers of such messages are seen as "outsiders" who have little appreciation of what actually goes on in the schools.)

Dr. C.: Were the reading scores for this school discussed?

Mr. J.: Yes, and I think we were all disappointed that the children hadn't improved more, but some gains were made. But coming back to what we were discussing, we thought that we would propose that you run a group counseling or group treatment session for these particular children, maybe once or maybe twice a week, and with the counselor watching so she could learn about it.

Dr. C.: Has the counselor been involved in planning for this?

Mr. J.: Oh yes, I discussed it with her and she's in complete agreement. She even volunteered to sit in with you. ("Volunteering" at a school is analogous to volunteering in the military; i.e., there are many ways of making someone do it.)

(The telephone rings again. The principal discusses with caller the problem of vandalism, and the need for iron grates on basement and first floor windows.)

Dr. C.:   You're very busy.

Mr. J.:   Yes, busy with things that don't have much to do with education. (Very true, he's a former teacher, probably was a very good one, and he now spends his time doing what he likes least.)

Dr. C.:   I was wondering, could I talk to the counselor, today?

Mr. J.:   Unfortunately, she's teaching a class now, filling in for one of our teachers who is sick.

Dr. C.:   Maybe I'll get to see her another time then. One more question. Was there any particular reason you called me now? Any sort of "last straw" that made you think that some mental health work might be useful?

Mr. J.:   Well, nothing specific. It just seems that the further we get in the school year, the worse it gets. And these children really do get to my teachers. Some of those teachers threatened to quit, but I don't think they mean it. We don't have as much trouble with the younger children.

Dr. C.:   I have a rough idea of the problem. Let me think about it and get back to you. I'll probably want to come back and meet with you again, with the counselor, and perhaps some of the teachers.

SELF-REFLECTION

On his way back to his office, Dr. C. asks himself the following questions:

1. Who's hurting? As far as I can tell, it's mainly the principal, and if he's right, also the teachers. I don't know the counselor's role in this yet and I really know very little about the children.
2. Why are they calling me now? The principal's last remark may be the most significant. He said a few teachers might quit, and he really seems pressured to do something. He wants to get the teachers off his back, maybe.
3. What is their current theory of the problem? It seems to be that it's mostly the children's fault. They probably do have some difficult children. But he also said Miss Taylor seems to have the most trouble and she's new. What about the way the other fifth and sixth grade teachers handle the problems? I should find out how he views the other teachers.

4. What might be camouflaged? Hard to say, but there might be a really
    big hassle between those teachers and the principal about some other
    things. The turnover rate is high, although not way out of line for city
    schools. It may be that overall morale is bad. There is also some hint
    that the teachers are frustrated with their effectiveness in helping
    children read. And even though the counselor had to fill in for another
    teacher, I don't think that the principal had invited her to our meeting
    anyway; nor does it sound as if he fully discussed it with her.
5. Is there a problem which could be helped by mental health input?
    Perhaps. I'd want to know more. Certainly, I want to talk to those
    other people. A group meeting with the teachers really might give me
    a better idea.
6. Do I want to get involved with this school and what are my personal
    priorities? I like the principal and have also heard that his reputation is
    good. Unless I can be convinced, however, I really don't want to work
    with the children in a group. I can do that kind of thing back at the
    clinic. If I'm going to work in the school, I'd rather work with school
    personnel than with the children. Maybe I could help people in the
    school to help other children. I'd like to at least go ahead and explore
    it with them.
7. What are my resources? If I work out a consultative program here, I'll
    have to do it alone. No one in my agency has the time to help me at
    this point. I don't like working alone but there is no other choice now.
    At least, I have the time available.

FURTHER EXPLORATION

Dr. C. meets with the counselor who says she is in agreement with the
principal's plan to establish a group therapy program for 12 children. She
has not had any experience in group counseling and is eager to learn from
Dr. C. He puts off that question for the time being and asks about her role
in the school. She is the only counselor for 600 children. In addition to
being overworked, she feels that her time is not always well used. Without
mentioning specific names, she indicates that certain teachers consider her
a disciplinarian and not a counselor. Children are sent to her when they are
in trouble in the classroom, and she is expected to "straighten them out."
Teachers do not refer children to her early enough but wait until they are
causing big problems. Some teachers do not understand that shy and in-
hibited children can have emotional problems too, and it is not just the
children with behavior problems who are in difficulty. She is generally cir-
cumspect about the teachers but feels that they "need help." She also

gently reminds the consultant that she tried to refer children to his clinic, but they have to wait at least several weeks for an appointment. Even after the child is seen, the school does not get very much feedback.

Next a meeting is arranged between Dr. C. and the fifth and sixth grade teachers, after clearance from the principal. The teachers are quite friendly and talkative.

Teacher #1: Are we glad to see you. Maybe we need our heads shrunk, not the kids. (Self-conscious laughter. Almost all teachers, when they first meet a mental health consultant, think that he is about to "analyze" them. If he really plans to do that, then he's in big trouble.)

Teacher #2: Yes, you'd have to be crazy to work here.

Dr. C.: Why?

Teacher #2: This really isn't a bad school as schools go, but it's awfully hard to keep some of these kids in line.

Teacher #3: The teachers are supposed to do everything, teach the kids, control them, babysit them, and then, as soon as something goes wrong, it's always the teacher's fault.

Dr. C.: Who blames you?

Teacher #1: I had a parent the other day who said his child was getting such bad grades because I wasn't teaching him right, she was going to go see Mr. J.

Teacher #4: Did she?

Teacher #1: I don't know. If she did, he didn't tell me about it.

Teacher #5 (to consultant abruptly): Do you have any experience with the open classroom?

Dr. C.: Some, in one of the schools I consulted before. Why?

Teacher #5: Well, we're trying to do it in some of the fifth grade classes, but we don't think it's working. If anything, it makes the children's behavior worse.

Teacher #3: These kids aren't ready for it. It may work out OK in some private schools, but not here.

Dr. C.: How did you get into the open classroom idea?

Teacher #5: It was the principal's idea, and I think he got it from the local district superintendent.

Teacher #3: It's in vogue, it's the thing to do.

Dr. C.: Did you get any training before you started?

Teacher #3: We had a part-time 4-week summer orientation course, and then we began. But it's like any other training. *Doing* it is something different and nobody around here seems to understand much about it.

Teacher #1:   From what I've seen, we know enough about it to know it won't work. We need more discipline around here, not less.

The discussion continues. The teachers complain about the behavior of some of the children, the lack of parental interest, problems of communication within the school, the lack of adequate supportive services. The sense of frustration is palpable and slightly overwhelming. Dr. C. comes away deluged with information about how teachers view life in their school.

RETHINKING AND TASK FORMULATION

After sorting out his observations about School XYZ, Dr. C. decides that he would like to develop a consultation program primarily involving the teachers, using the Teacher Discussion Model described below. His plan is to work with teachers in a group to achieve the following:

1. To develop a mutual support system within the group so that teachers might plan and work together more effectively;
2. To encourage communication between this group and the principal;
3. To develop behavioral management techniques after discussion with the group and to implement those in the classroom; and
4. Hopefully to increase staff morale through the successful achievement of items 1, 2, and 3.

How he will specifically accomplish these objectives is not clear in his mind, but is dependent on future meetings which he wishes to have with the teachers. He has a rough outline, however, and he now shares it with the principal.

RENEGOTIATION (OR CONTINUING NEGOTIATION)

After Dr. C. reports on his observations and explains his plan to the principal, the following dialogue ensues:

Mr. J.:   This plan really doesn't involve any group work with the children, but just the teachers.

Dr. C.:   That's right. I think maybe I can have more of an impact on the whole fifth or sixth grade program if I work this way. Maybe we can cut down on the number of disruptive children if the teachers feel more confident and can manage their classes more effectively.

Mr. J.: I'm a bit skeptical that the teachers will really let you in on that kind of thing. After all, you're an outsider. It's going to take some hard work with the teachers.

Dr. C.: I know. I'd have to work out more details of the program with them.

Mr. J.: There's another problem. The teachers can't stay after school for these meetings unless they are paid. We don't have any money to do that. If they meet just once a week with you during the school day, it means getting substitutes to cover their classes. Unless you want to meet over lunch, which is 45 minutes long and kind of noisy. I'll have to look into these things and get back to you. Your idea might be worth a try. The teachers could use some help. (The objections Mr. J. raises seem realistic, but do they really cover up his underlying resistance?)

Dr. C.: You let me know whether these meetings are possible, and then I can begin meeting with the teachers.

Mr. J.: Oh, by the way, the meetings with the teachers will probably take 1 to 1.5 hours. But if you're going to be here about a morning or afternoon a week, could you occasionally see a problem child and discuss his problems with us?

Dr. C.: (Feeling somewhat hemmed in but willing to compromise.) Yes, I suppose I could do that from time to time, but I really do want to spend most of my time with the teachers.

Mr. J.: Of course, I'll look into it and get back to you.

And so it begins.

In this particular example, the request came from the school. The consultant responded and a plan was elaborated after a series of meetings. What if the initial request had been made by the consultant, who then went to the school to "sell" them on the idea? Some of the negotiation is similar to the above school-initiated request but the differences are highlighted in Chapter 11 in the discussion on the Incentive Specialist Program. In Chapter 11 we will also consider other issues relevant to the later stages of a school consultation program, for example, maintenance, termination, and evaluation.

Some pertinent and vital questions have either been neglected or inadequately highlighted in the above dialogue. When the negotiation process begins between principal and consultant, the consultant may not always ask a key question, "Is there any money available?" If there is not, then he must consider whether the program can be undertaken at all, given that it would mean some reordering of clinic priorities and the withdrawal of services from one particular area to give to another area. Being faced with such a decision may be quite useful in the sense that the mental health professional then tends to reflect more about what the future direction of his own clinic should be. But too often, in our experience, clinics have offered services free, out of a sense of interest and public service, without imposing enough responsibility on the schools for providing or finding funds. In our economic society, services that are paid for are more valued than services that are not paid for. Fees impose the obligation on both the service giver and the service receiver of evaluating the worth of those services.

The question of money, however, is only one of the obstacles in the negotiating process. Frequently, it becomes clear that the principal is requesting a program which will not involve him. He may have decided that he wants to develop a special education class, or that he wants a consultant to work with a group of remedial teachers, or with his school counselors. The principal may present himself as someone, however, who has already "seen the light" and for whom consultation services are not really necessary. (We do not mean to imply that only school principals may adopt this lofty attitude; mental health professionals, too, when they go into a school may see themselves more as teachers than learners, and both roles are essential if any program is to succeed.) It is probably obvious to all of us now that any program which does not actively involve the school principal stands a good chance of being doomed to failure, just as individual work with children, divorced from the family contact, may be fruitless. Furthermore, the principal and consultant may each adopt the "father knows best" attitude, and the very people (teachers, counselors, parents, home and school coordinators, and even pupils) with whom most of the collaborative work will be done may be excluded from these early meetings. A contract is worked out between the bosses and the program is presented to the workers. Chances for sabotage using such an approach are limitless and highly probable.

Other essential points basic to the program may be overlooked: What room will the consultant use? Will it always be available or will he wander, gypsylike, from week to week? Does the consultant get a parking space in the school parking lot? Will teachers always be available at a specified time, and are there plans for adequate classroom coverage? Will the school be open at night if parents' meetings are a part of the program? What is the procedure for resolving the above difficulties? And finally, a fundamental question: Are there any evaluative procedures built into the program from the beginning so that some notion of success or failure can be objectified?

In a particularly compelling paper, Berkovitz[1] "tells it like it is" in his description of the problems involved in setting up and maintaining school consultation programs. He stresses the need to attend carefully to such issues as power, sanction, overt and covert expectations, and the maintenance of relationships with school administrative personnel.

Ruth Newman[2] has advocated an open-ended approach which

prolongs the whole negotiating process and may ensure a higher acceptance rate between school and consultant. She feels that the consultant should be given a lengthy, free-time period at the beginning to give him an opportunity to "nose around"; to chat with teachers and others at lunch; and to get a feel for the school climate and its problems before any definite plans are made to work with a particular sector or issue. This approach, comparable to an extended diagnostic evaluation of a family, is desirable, but may be too luxurious for consultants and schools who want to "get something done."

MODELS OF SCHOOL CONSULTATION

Let us now examine what "gets done." We will consider five models of school consultation. Although the models are apparently typical of the interventions that are currently being attempted, we also realize that there are different approaches that will not be covered.

Special Classroom Model

In this model the psychiatrist or psychologist serves as the consultant to a special class teacher and counselor. Children referred to the special class generally have learning or behavior disabilities, or both, and tend to remain in special class placement for 1 to 2 years. The consultant evaluates individual children, meets regularly with the teacher and counselor, may conduct parent or children's groups, and, in general, seeks to apply his psychological knowledge to problems of individual children and to strategies of classroom management. Although this model may give some children "breathing time" in a small classroom setting with a compassionate teacher, it does pose some noteworthy disadvantages. Children placed in the class tend to consider themselves "dumb" or "bad"; the consultant may add an additional label, that of being "sick." Often the children, teacher, and even the consultant feel isolated from the rest of the school program, and this isolation may be reinforced by the unconscious exclusion of the special class participants by the rest of the school. Special class placement may become a one-way street; it can be used as a dumping ground for difficult children, and resistances are mobilized once it is time to return one of these children to his regular class. And finally, there are no conclusive studies showing that special class placement for children with emotional disturbances is beneficial academically, although there is perhaps some evidence that it is of use in terms of improving behavior. By now it has certainly been relatively well documented that special class placement for the overwhelming majority of retarded children is not indicated.[3]

One particular modification of special class placement merits attention and apparently has produced beneficial results. Glavin et al.[4] have used a behavior therapy approach in a "resource room" setting, in which a token economy system is used for children who spend most of their day in a regular class placement.

The Teacher Discussion Model

This model generally involves group discussion between teachers and consultant about various mental health principles, such as early identification, hyperactivity, the withdrawn child, and techniques of classroom management. (In terms of the latter point, we offer a caveat: most consultants know very little about classrooms, have rarely been in a classroom, have been trained primarily to work with individual children rather than with groups, and feel that questions of curriculum may be irrelevant.) Our experience with such teacher discussion groups indicates that the first few sessions may be spent on the problem of "What should we do about Johnny who won't sit still in his seat?" However, the teachers soon move on to other areas of concern which are even more vital to their interest. Teachers, like some of their pupils, frequently feel frustrated, alone, and inadequate. The presence of a consultant may serve as a catalyst for their complaints and frustrations. They soon begin talking about problems between the teachers, between the teachers and the administration, about ratings from their supervisors, about who eats lunch with the principal and who does not, about the cliques in the school, about the problems of new teachers in the system, about the "relevance" of the curriculum, and about their pervasive feeling of impotence. Verbalization, like love, however, is not enough.

A consultant may feel awkward in such meetings because he has never really developed a contract to pursue the agenda that the group is developing. Equally important, the group sees itself as not having power to change anything in the system; and in truth, it has not received sanction to do anything but talk, and perhaps learn. The teachers in the group, again like their pupils, can be confronted with a troublesome environment, but the group is not offered the tools with which they can alter their destiny. Our impression is that such discussion groups are workable only if the group, as a group, can work on some directed activity which intimately affects their professional lives in the school. For instance, a group of seventh grade teachers might be offered the opportunity to develop a new math curriculum, or a Black Studies Program, or any project which they and their pupils could feel was their own. The issues and conflicts that arise out of such a venture could then be effectively used in a group discussion format that would present more of a "real life" experience aimed at growth and not just shared complaints and frustrations.

One of the authors (M. Forman), together with two other mental health professionals, were members of a teacher discussion group which adopted a task-oriented approach. The group felt that the gap between parents and schools represented a significant obstacle in their work with children. The teachers rarely met parents of the students, except in a crisis situation when defenses on both sides were mobilized. The discussion group, with all members participating, decided that a home-visiting project might help narrow the parent-school distance. The consultants assisted the group in designing a training workshop in home-visit preparation and techniques. After an initial period of role playing in which mental health personnel and teachers both simulated parents and visiting teachers, pairs of discussion group members began visiting homes of children. Generally, a mental health professional and a teacher made the home visits together. Each wrote down his observation independently following the visit, and then both reported back to the total group. Issues relating to observational discrepancies, socioeconomic differences and biases, teacher expectations, and parental suspiciousness soon emerged and provided more than ample "live" material for the discussion group. Even more important, the teachers felt that they were doing something "real," and that they had gained some understanding of the home lives of their pupils which was related to their classroom performance. And because of the home-visit training experience which the mental health consultants provided, the teachers now had another technique in their repertoire which they could carry on after the consultants left.

Classroom Discussion Model

The foremost proponents of this particular style of school intervention are Kellam and Schiff,[5] formerly of the Woodlawn Community Mental Health Center in Chicago. In a series of papers, they describe the approach to the selection of the community, the basic elements of the program, the evaluation design, and the results. They particularly stress the importance of gaining sanction from recognized groups within the community, specifying the type of population and its needs, and carrying out programs in an appropriate social context. Their negotiations with the empowered community organization led to a mutual decision that mental health intervention would be directed at all first graders in the schools of the community. The goals of intervention were to promote and maintain adaptation to the tasks of first grade. The method involved classroom discussions conducted by the consultant and teacher once a week and several times weekly by the teacher alone. Questions usually centered around the theme, "What do you have to do to make it in first grade?" Comments on the behavior of their peers were made by students; parents were invited by students to join the classroom discussion, and were also involved in additional parent meetings. This program has been an extraordinarily well-designed research endeavor, and the reports have indicated some beneficial effects in the experimental groups. The approach is somewhat similar to that described by Bronfenbrenner[6] in his book, "The Two Worlds of Childhood: U.S. and U.S.S.R.," in which he recounts numerous anecdotes of classroom discussions in Soviet schools in which the norms of peer group behavior were emphasized in discussions between teachers and pupils. A much earlier paper by Levy[7] recounts his experiences visiting classrooms in Vienna in which the students and teachers were in active dialogue about their behavior, using Adlerian psychology as a basis for discussion.

Using his "reality therapy and approach," Glasser[8] has evolved another technique of daily classroom discussions led by the teacher. These can be of three types: (1) social problem-solving meetings; (2) open-ended meetings concerned with intellectually important subjects; and (3) educational diagnostic meetings focused on how well the students understand the concepts of the curriculum. Glasser urges that these meetings become incorporated as a part of the regular school curriculum, and particularly stresses that the meetings be oriented toward solving a problem and should never result in punishment or blame. He gives numerous anecdotes and examples from his personal experience in the use of this technique with children of elementary and high school age. In this situation, the consultant serves as teacher for a group of teachers. The teachers are then free to develop their own styles in implementing the principles of the classroom meeting. The consultant observes and suggests and helps the teacher refine the technique and deal with problems encountered.

Educators are more likely to develop programs based on this model. We suspect that the mental health consultant feels more exposed in dealing with the teacher and class in vivo than he does in the models discussed previously. It may also be difficult to accept the notion that young children can talk in a classroom about classroom problems, but it is also quite likely that they are rarely given the opportunity to do so.

Community Intervention Model

There are few reports of community intervention although Wahler and Erickson[9] described the activities of public health nurses and trained professional volunteers who used behavioral reinforcement techniques in classroom situations to modify disruptive behavior. However, this model implies a more general strategy related to mental health and social institutions in a community. Schools are located within communities, but their dealings with each other primarily have been in terms of the trafficking of children. The school as an integral social force playing a responsible and mutually enhancing role with a community in which it exists is a relatively rare phenomenon. Schools share with other social institutions the general alienation from populations they were established to serve.

One such attempt to bridge the gap between the community and the school is the program developed by the Young Great Society, a black community self-help group, and the Temple Community Mental Health Center in Philadelphia.[10] In collaboration with the public schools, and specifically some junior high schools in the catchment area, the center has devised a program of classroom intervention using paraprofessionals who are designated as "incentive specialists." The incentive specialists are black adults, male or female, in their early twenties. They are recruited and trained by the staff of the Young Great Society and the mental health center. Their role is an educationally enhancing one. The program is deemed a positive mental health intervention, and it is not an identification of ill, handicapped, or disturbed children. The specialist works with the children around the achievement of educational goals and serves as an overall model. He establishes a working contract with the classroom teacher, and serves as a communication bridge through which that teacher can reach her children. (See Chapter 11 for a full discussion of this program.)

The mental health consultant further serves as a psychiatric consultant for individual children when their emotional problems, behavior, or learning difficulties become too significantly puzzling, difficult, or complex for the specialist or the other school staff. All precautions are taken in this consultation procedure to gain the full confidence and participation of the parents and to reassure both parents and other community members, as well as teachers, that the psychiatrist is not there to label children as ill and thus justify their exclusion from school.

The project has a strong built-in research evaluative component in which intervention and control classes are compared, using such variables as grades, disciplinary actions, attendance, suspensions, migration in and out of the classroom, as well as some specially designed instruments to evaluate the attitudes of both children and teaching staff.

"Crash Program" Model

Finally, there is another kind of school consultation program which is characterized more by circumstances in which it occurs, rather than by any

one specific intervention technique. The methods applied may be those applied in any of the other models, but the form of entry differs.

Occasionally, mental health personnel are drawn into schools in a
crisis situation in which the schools perceive that "something" must be
done quickly. Funding is usually immediately available, since the crisis
may be related to some disruption which has communitywide effects, for
example, gangs, racial turmoil, drug abuse. Mental health personnel are
viewed as being problem solvers of the crisis, though the roots of the
difficulty may be far removed from their expertise and influence. In the
rush to get a crash program underway, the niceties of the negotiation
process previously elaborated are ignored. The consultant may find
himself confronted with political and administrative realities which prede-
termine his role, limit his functions, and frustrate his efforts.

To illustrate, we review the development of the "School Discipline
Team," a program enacted in February of 1969 in 21 of Philadelphia's
secondary schools.[11] Before describing the purposes and composition of
these ill-named teams, we must first identify some of the major social and
political issues which led to their development.

In Philadelphia, there had been a long-standing feud between the current and former mayors, the latter serving in 1969 as the president of the
School Board of Education. The chronic financial crisis made the schools
an easy target for the mayor and the party in power, whose support was
needed for school bond issues which did not always pass. Previous attempts had been made by the city administration to gain control of the
school district budget and patronage positions.

Added to this power struggle of some years' duration, there was
increasing racial unrest in schools in the community. A large and peaceful
demonstration by black students requesting a black history course was
brutally repressed by the police in front of the school administration
building. Consequently, serious riots erupted in several secondary schools.
Public reaction was immediate and polarized around the law and order
theme. This response was exploited in an election year when the city machine wished to deliver a large plurality for its favorite presidential candidate. The mayor stated that his first concern was "the alleviation of fear in
the community" and proposed a series of measures which included: (1) the
establishment of detention centers for disruptive children; (2) stationing of
police within schools; (3) transfer of the school budget to the city; and (4)
abandonment of plans for decentralization.

A group of mental health professionals submitted formal objections
to these proposals and offered counter suggestions. These suggestions
generally stressed the need for small leadership groups in the schools, composed of community representatives, faculty, students, administration, and
mental health personnel. These teams were to look at the school "cli-

mate," to investigate relationships between school and community and intraschool relationships which influenced learning, and to develop crisis-intervention techniques for problem situations in schools. These proposals appeared to be acceptable to the school district, but during the negotiation process, school administrators changed their stance and submitted a different proposal to city administration. These teams were now to be called "School Discipline Teams," which could recommend transfer of students, filing of delinquency petitions, or the arrest of certain individual pupils. The schools had offered City Council a politically palatable program which said "Hands off, we can be tough, too."

City Council then appropriated the funds for these teams and they were on their way. Mental health personnel were invited to join *after* school principals had already hand-picked the teachers, students, and community representatives. The function of the mental health members, as defined by the principals and the teams, was to be primarily that of screening and testing individual "sick" or "bad" children, some of whom were being referred to "vestibule" special classes within the school.

Given this disarray, it is quite logical to ask the question, "Why did the mental health consultants ever agree to join such a venture?" Do consultants participate in a poorly designed, hastily conceived program with the hope of changing the situation and altering objectives, or do they refuse outright? We accepted the invitation for the following reasons:

1. It was better than having police in the schools.
2. We did not want to superimpose our preconceived ideas on the schools.
3. We had a good relationship with the local district superintendent, although these teams were more clearly the responsibility of the local school principals.
4. Probably the most glorious rationalization of all, we wanted to learn something.

What happened once the teams began in these 21 schools? Not much. From the beginning, the teams did not have clear-cut authority to do anything. The principal usually called the shots but rarely came to meetings. The teams were also under pressure to produce and felt the need to have concrete projects underway rather than to give attention to the process by which schools and teams operated. The teams, too, tended to be polarized around the law and order theme, without any resolution. Funds ran out in 3 months and no one knew whether they would be available for the next academic year. The few schools in which teams did some effective work were good schools in which interesting programs had developed before the advent of the teams. None of the teams is in existence today after an expenditure of more than 1 million dollars.

SUMMARY

Using a pragmatic point of view, we have attempted to delineate potential sources of conflict between schools and consultants, with particular emphasis on the initial negotiation process. We have described models of consultation, not with the intention of presenting recipes for every occasion, but rather to illustrate the variety of approaches that have evolved, as well as their merits and deficiencies. We realize that we are open to the charge of being "too negative," of citing hindrances without proposing positive steps.

We know that we are being critical of the ways schools operate. Schools are an easy target, however, and we could probably have been equally critical of the methods of consultants who too often pose as fuzzy-minded experts who patronize school personnel. As Mark Twain said, "Being good is noble; teaching others to be good is nobler, and no trouble."

Our own experience leads us to believe that because of mutual dissatisfaction between educators and consultants, there may be fewer viable consultation programs now than there were several years ago. Perhaps, a recitation of pitfalls may have an educational value for the readers, and at least a therapeutic value for the authors. Given that school consultation has become a serious area of commitment for school personnel, we hope that further efforts will be directed at clarifying the purposes of our interventions and the success or failure of our efforts.

Finally, the following propositions are presented in the imperative mode. They are offered in the manner of a Baedeker to simplify survival in a foreign land. In some, equally battle-scarred, they may find a responsive chord and form the basis of consensus or dispute. For the novice to school consultation, they serve the same functions as all maxims, rules, commandments, advice, proverbs, and hoary utterances—an opportunity to thumb one's nose. These rules are offered without elaboration, since to do justice to each one would require another chapter:

1. Get trained in consultation first, or else begin by working with an experienced consultant.
2. Be clear about what you have in mind to do, remembering that the crucial decisions affect the ingredients of people, time, space, and money.
3. You should know and visit your principal regularly.
4. Take your time in reaching a final plan for your program.
5. Be stubborn about any change in your program once it has begun.
6. Do not work alone.

7. Find allies in the school; know why they are allies.
8. Be a good maintenance person: careful attention to administrative trivia can mean the difference between the success or failure of a program.
9. Keep a log or a journal.
10. Have full support of your sponsoring agency or group.
11. Evaluate. You must plan it in advance.
12. And finally, to end on a less pessimistic note, keep in mind the maxim of the May 1967 French Student Rebellion: "The best people work only for lost causes, realizing that the others are merely effects."

REFERENCES

1. Berkovitz IH: Mental health consultation to school personnel: attitudes of school administrators and consultant priorities. J School Health 40:348–354, 1970
2. Newman RG: Psychological Consultation in the Schools. New York, Basic Books, 1967
3. Sarason SB, Doris J: Psychological Problems in Mental Deficiency (ed 4). New York, Harper & Row, 1969
4. Glavin JP, Quay HC, Werry JS: Behavioral and academic gains of conduct problem children in different classroom settings. Except Child 37:441–446, 1971
5. Kellam S, Schiff S: Adaptation and mental illness in the first grade classrooms of an urban community. Psychiat Res Rep 21: 79–91, 1967
6. Bronfenbrenner U: The Two Worlds of Childhood: U.S. and U.S.S.R. New York, Russel Sage Foundation, 1970
7. Levy DM: "Individual psychology" in a Vienna public school. Soc Serv Rev 3:207–216, 1929
8. Glasser W: Schools Without Failure. New York, Harper & Row, 1969
9. Wahler RG, Erickson M: Child behavior therapy: a community program in Appalachia. Behav Res Ther 7:71–78, 1969
10. Hetznecker W, Bruce D: The role of a community mental health center as a mediator between school and community. Paper presented at annual meeting of American Psychiatric Association, Miami, Florida, 1969
11. Forman M, Glass A: School discipline team: destination unknown. Paper presented at annual meeting of American Association of Psychiatric Services for Children, Boston, Massachusetts, 1969

L. Wayne Higley
Bari Blumenstein

6

The Day Diagnostic Center

THE PROBLEM

One of the questions most frequently asked of mental health consultants who were collaborating with school personnel was, "How do I deal with this child in the classroom?" We were usually able to acquire some understanding of the underlying dynamics of a child's behavior, his strengths and weaknesses, and his general learning style. We could generally put together some picture of the child in relation to his particular environment: family, neighborhood, school. Out of this understanding we could often make some hypotheses about his classroom functioning, and devise some proposals for the school's response to him.

But such proposals were often received with little enthusiasm by the school personnel, and were often ignored or even subverted. Although the analyses and prescriptions prepared by consulting clinical staff might be quite perceptive and appropriate, they were rarely based on direct experience in teaching a child in a group situation, a fact which teachers were quick to spot and exploit. This was particularly true when the prescription called for changes in the child's school program instead of referral for treatment at the clinic. School personnel wanted the clinic to do "something" with the *child,* at the *clinic,* not "something" with the *teacher,* at the *school.* In response to this, clinical personnel perceived rejection of the child, and tended to focus on the inability of the school to accept alternatives. School personnel began to question the clinical skill (if not the motives) of the consultant; clinical personnel became angry at the school as a rigid, inadequate system. The ultimate result was all too often the deterioration of school-clinic relationships.

Recognizing that clinical personnel did not, in fact, have an opportunity to experience teaching and managing children in groups, we sensed that we needed to extend and verify our understanding and prescriptions by actually working with children as students in groups.

THE PLAN

This persistent problem led us to the conception of the Day Diagnostic Center. Note that, as with many innovations, the form of our "solution" was greatly affected by the fortuitous availability of space. Several large rooms adjacent to the clinic waiting room became vacant. In this space we determined to work out some of the solutions to our consultation problems. One room was outfitted as a classroom for 8 to 10 children. A wide variety of materials and equipment were purchased, with special attention to those which lent themselves to individualized teaching and self-programming. The classroom was directed by a therapeutic teacher who had had experience as an activities therapist in a psychiatric setting. She was assisted by an aide, and the entire program was placed under the supervision of an educational psychologist who also had had experience in special education. We planned that a child's primary therapist would be closely involved during a child's stay in the DDC and in subsequent work with his school. A major job of the DDC would be working with the schools to which children returned and, therefore, we added the role of liaison counselor to assure that function.[1] The liaison counselor would become thoroughly informed about the findings and recommendations of the DDC. She would follow-up the child in his community school as long as necessary to assist the teacher in putting into operation new teaching strategies and materials. Administratively the DDC was part of the Children & Family Unit of the Mental Health Center (see Chap. 3).

We did not try to reproduce the child's usual school situation. A child would attend the DDC for some portion of or all of his school day, for periods up to 3 weeks, only long enough for the therapeutic teacher to determine the child's responses to group situations and to various learning expectations and teaching strategies. An observation room was built so that the therapist, classroom teacher, and other concerned persons (including parents) could increase their understanding of the child's behavior by watching him function in a group-learning situation.

Referrals were to be initiated by center therapists, classroom teachers, and school counselors through the liaison counselor. Eligibility was limited to 8 to 10-year-old's who were considered to be unmanageable in school. We were particularly interested in children who were excluded from school on psychiatric grounds, who were regularly suspended, or who presented combinations of retardation and dysfunctional behavior. The liaison counselor would observe the child in his own classroom, paying attention to his learning and behavior assets and liabilities. His teacher was asked to fill out a learning and behavioral checklist. The liaison counselor

Table 6.1
Sex, Age, Grade and Presenting Problems of 10 Children
Referred to Day Diagnostic Program

Student	Sex	Age	Grade	Presenting Problems
Joe	M	9–7	Not attending (later placed in RT class	Excluded from school because of failure to learn and behavior
Chris	M	11-12	5th	Reading below grade level
Sam	M	10–10	5th	Behavior problem; academic work two grades behind
Gloria	F	10–1	4th	Very slow, working below rest of class
Bill	M	10–11	RE	Reading at primer level; can not follow directions
Charles	M	9–7	Middle house at intensive learning center	Seems to be "lost" all the time; works below other children in group; what instructional techniques should be used?
Ron	M	8–1	2nd	Hyperactive, inattentive, work sometimes good, sometimes terrible
Bruce	M	10–5	4th	Fighting; talks out in class, can do more work when he tries; what motivates him?
Mark	M	12–1	RE	Does not participate in class; reading much above other skills which are below level of class
Brian	M	10–10	5th	Plays around in class, can do work when wants to; teacher thinks might be too bright for present class

interviewed parents to obtain information about family interaction, discipline methods used at home, and parents' perceptions of the child's school problems. If a child was accepted into the DDC, he would become a client of the center and in most cases his family was to be involved in treatment.

The DDC room was arranged to delineate four learning areas: language, conceptual, perceptual, and social.[2-5] Activities were scheduled so that each child had an opportunity to work and be observed in each learning area each day. Materials and activities were selected to encourage each child to make use of a number of different situations and learning modalities, thus enabling the teacher to determine the child's particular strengths and weaknesses. The total emphasis was on finding those specific expectations to which the child could respond positively, and the techniques and materials which worked best for him. Daily sessions were scheduled from 9:30 to 2:30, with children attending for varying portions of the day. A typical day's schedule follows:

9:30–10:00: *Language.* This included work in language development skills such as vocabulary, written and verbal expression, articulation, spelling, listening comprehension. These activities as well as those that follow were usually done individually or in small groups. Seldom was the entire DDC class working on the same material at the same time.

10:00–10:30: *Arithmetic.* Activities were designed to explore the child's ability with basic number concepts, counting, and understanding of sets.

10:30–10:45: *Break.* (snack)

10:45–11:00: *Perceptual skills.* Experiences in both visual and auditory perception were given. Included were activities for identifying sounds, following directions, understanding of what was seen or heard, memory for oral and visual information, generally and in a sequence, organization and manipulating of visual symbols, and oral information.

11:00–11:30: *Reading.* Assigned in this area were work attack skills, recognition of component parts of words, phonetic association, sound blending, number and kinds of errors (substitution omissions, insertions) made when reading. The Fernald Method (Verbal Auditory Kinesthetic, Tactile) was sometimes tried to determine its effectiveness as a reading approach.

11:30–11:45: *Independent activity.* Activity might be a game or teacher prepared worksheet or work at a learning center. The period allowed the teacher to observe the child's work habits, how tasks were approached, motivation, concentration.

11:45–12:00: *Perceptual skill*

12:00–1:00: *Lunch and outdoor recess (games)*

1:00–1:30: *Cognitive skills.* These included sorting, categorizing, labeling, and availability of general information, i.e., current events, geography, knowledge of the community.

1:30–2:00: *Group projects (arts and crafts).* The teacher was able to observe the children in a group situation. The projects were selected so that success depended on each child cooperating and doing his part of the work.

2:00–2:20: *Social skills.* Topics such as consequences of child's behavior and possible alternative behavior were discussed. Children were taught to role play problem situations and solutions.

2:20–2:30: *Cleanup and discussion of schedule for following day.*

Instructional Materials*

Language
  Peabody Language Development Kit
  Dolch Program and Games
  Educational Password
  Dolch Basic Sight Vocabulary
  Language Experience in Reading
  Listen and Do
  Reading Road to Spelling
Arithmetic
  Greater Cleveland Math Series
  Cuisenaire Rods
  Counting Games
  Number Line
  Number Steps
  Lotto
  Number Concepts
  U.S. Money
Perceptual
  Fitzhugh Program
  TRY
  Listening to Sounds
  Reading Thinking Series
  Frostig Program
  Dominoes
  Perception Cards
  Pegboard and Pegs
  Buzzer Board
  Independent Activities

*Detailed descriptions of these instructional materials and their use can be found in references 2 and 3.

Reading
  Sullivan Programmed Reading Series
  Dolch Program
  Phonics Drill Cards
  Word Wheels
  Records
  Beginning Sounds
  Quizmo
Conceptual
  Learning to Think Series
Social
  Basic Social Studies Discussion
  Pictures
  Stories

The teacher and the aide kept detailed observational records. A psychologist, psychiatrist, and educational specialist were also available to provide additional evaluative information if indicated. Specific diagnostic procedures were tailored to each child; no routine battery of tests was predetermined. Assessment procedures were to be built around very specific questions as they were formulated.

During the diagnostic period, the child's classroom teacher, school counselor, and center therapist were encouraged to visit the DDC and observe the child they had referred. We hoped that by viewing the child in a learning environment designed to accommodate to his learning and behavior style, the teacher might revise her attitude toward the child and her teaching techniques when dealing with the child in his regular classroom. At the end of each child's stay in the DDC, a psychoeducational prescription was prepared using learning and behavioral information gathered by the DDC personnel. Formal testing results provided by the psychologist and educational specialist, and pertinent information gathered from parents were included. The psychoeducational analysis and prescription included four parts.

1. The teacher's perception of the child and formal test results. This section included informatiuon on child's reaction to other children in the DDC, and to the teacher and aide, his reinforcement patterns, his work habits, defenses used by the child, and significant test results. A typical entry in this section might be: "John sits alone and seldom plays with the other children. He is not able to admit that he cannot do or that he does not know. Instead he tries to divert the teacher's attention by hitting others or throwing things. He is of below average intelligence as measured by the WISC; however, there is a wide spread among subtest scores." (These scores are then detailed and interpreted.)

2. Needs of the child. Examples from this section include: "John has difficulty associating the sound of a word with the visual symbol. His auditory memory is one of his weakest learning abilities. He is unable to recall more than four numbers. John relies on pictures to help him comprehend what he is reading."

3. Specific techniques and materials useful in meeting the child's needs. This section contained a list of recommended materials and their uses. Materials suggested might include specific programmed materials, prepackaged kits as well as specific series. Teaching techniques such as VAKT, specific reading methods, and materials that are reinforcers were also recommended when necessary.

4. How to plan and organize classroom activities so that the materials and methods can be used in the classroom. Suggestions were given for classroom organization designed to accommodate the use of prescribed materials and techniques. Typical recommendations include: "John appears apprehensive in new learning situations. Consistency in daily scheduling is needed so that he will know what is expected of him in each situation. Work to be done should be presented in small segments and clearly defined. A 'programmed series' should be used." (Examples are suggested.)

The complete psychoeducation prescription with specific recommendations was to be relayed to the classroom teacher through the liaison counselor. The liaison counselor would discuss the prescription with the classroom teacher, answer questions, and actively support the teacher over a period of time. Materials which had been recommended but were not available to the teachers were to be provided. The liaison counselor and the teacher would discuss any problems that arose as a result of implementing the recommendations in the classroom and offer suggestions for the next steps in remediating the child's learning difficulties or dealing with behavior problems.

EARLY CHANGES IN PROGRAM

As originally conceived, the target population for the DDC was to be primarily those children in the center caseload who had been excluded or frequently suspended from school because of serious learning or behavior problems, or both. The DDC was seen as an additional service which could be used by the therapist as part of a total treatment plan. In particular, we hoped that intervention by the DDC would increase the therapists' effectiveness in collaborating with the schools around a child's school program and management. Soon it became evident that center staff could not provide enough referrals to use the service fully.

In retrospect it seems we had overestimated the incidence of such cases. We also discovered that the purpose of the DDC was not fully understood and appreciated by center personnel. When they did turn to the DDC with a particular case, therapists considered this a referral from their caseload to that of the DDC, with a concomitant shift of full responsibility. The DDC was seen as an alternative rather than an adjunctive service.

In order to obtain information about children who fitted the DDC profile, the organizers of the DDC met with members of the School District. This channel for referrals was also blocked, primarily because of legal problems involving issues of confidentiality.

Therefore, in order to identify an alternative source of referrals, the DDC staff made contact with some schools, arranging for them to make direct referrals to the DDC through the liaison counselor. Children were not necessarily assigned to an outpatient therapist when accepted into the DDC. The DDC began to evolve into a discrete service of the center, with its own intake, treatment, and discharge procedures. This change stimulated alterations in the basic operations of the DDC and its personnel.

One result was a shift in the definition of the "appropriate case." Teachers and counselors (rather than center staff) became the primary referring agents. They were most interested in children whom they felt should be learning, but who were not. Fewer and fewer serious behavior problems were referred or accepted. Instead of serving children with serious behavior problems, the DDC became a program for children with complex learning problems.

By the time the DDC had begun, the center had gained the reputation of vigorous advocacy for keeping children in their community schools, and invoking all available supportive and remedial services within the school. We saw the schools as more capable than they thought they were. We did not readily take children off their hands by referring them to institutions. In fact, we knew that many children who were excluded or frequently suspended never received the full services and support of the school's special resources. In a surprising number of cases, such children were not even well known to counselors. These children were viewed by administrators as beyond the efforts of counselors, as just plain "bad actors." Their parents were or appeared to be so uncooperative as to make any effort useless, except repeated suspensions or other forms of threat. Given its traditional stance, the center was not seen as very helpful with such children since we did not usually support their removal from school or community.

Thus, at least three forces joined to change the definition of target population. Center personnel did not (for one reason or another) use the

DDC for their most difficult children; school personnel did not think of the center or the DDC as an appropriate resource; and the DDC, having developed its own intake function, did as most such services do—it worked with the most potentially successful cases, selecting learning problems rather than serious behavior problems.

As the target population changed, the function of various DDC personnel also changed. The liaison counselor became responsible for carrying out intake procedures for the increasing numbers of cases which did not come through other outpatient services. She spent a great deal more of her time on initial work-ups, observing children in school, gathering case histories, and dealing with school referral procedures. This meant that she had less time to work with DDC staff and to understand their findings and prescriptions. Most important, she had less opportunity to follow the child after his return to his classroom, and to give direction and support to his teacher.

As it became a discreet service with its own intake, the DDC routinely carried out its own mental health evaluations. Such procedures were necessarily time consuming, with reports coming so long after the initial inquiry that the DDC could no longer be viewed as a quick, short-term intervention. Inevitably, this further discouraged center therapists from using the DDC as part of a total treatment plan and further diminished the number of referrals coming through that route. They complained that reports took too long to be useful in dealing with children in school crises.

FOLLOW-UP

By the end of the school term, approximately 30 children had received psychoeducational evaluation in the DDC.

Follow-up of a small number (10) of the children was conducted through observation in the referring teacher's classroom and through conferences with the referring teacher to elicit her responses to the following:

1. Usefulness of the psychoeducational prescription.
2. Specific recommendations used.
3. Additions and modifications needed to make the prescription more usable.

The follow-up occurred at 1- and 3-month intervals after the prescription was delivered to the referring teacher. One month after the prescriptions were received, 4 of the 10 teachers stated that they had tried some of the prescriptive recommendations and were observed using the activities and materials in the classroom. These teachers found the prescriptions useful because "recommendations were specific and presented in educational terms rather than in unfamiliar psychological jargon." Two teachers said that provision of otherwise unavailable materials was the selling point for the prescription. The recommended activities used most frequently were those designed to remediate visual-perceptual deficits. The teachers found these activities were the easiest to fit into the classroom schedule (probably because the child could work on these independently). The remaining six teachers had not attempted to use any of the recommended materials and activities for a variety of reasons:

I wasn't trained to deal with a child who has special learning problems. I'm not an expert and shouldn't be expected to give individualized work in my classroom. These children belong in a special class.

The liaison counselor was another person who came to my classroom to add more work to my already overcrowded schedule.

The recommendation might have been useful if I had a full-time aide to help in the classroom. I just did not have time to try the recommendation myself.

If I refer a child to a place that tells me I should be able to accommodate the child's learning needs in my own classroom, it sounds as if there's something wrong with my teaching.

The principal says I have to follow the teacher's guide. This is third grade and the children should be doing academic work at this level and not doing puzzles or reading a primer.

I wanted to find out how to stop the behavior outbursts, not what and how to teach.

I was already using materials and activities similar to the ones recommended.

After 3 months, three of the four teachers who were using the recommendations continued to do so. (None of the other six teachers began to make use of the recommendations). All three who were following recommendations were special education teachers. The three teachers stated that the activities and materials recommended in the prescription were similar to those they were using in their classrooms.

The teachers suggested the following modifications: more information concerning the child's family situation, more specific "how to" methods for dealing with behavior problems, more frequent and longer visits by liaison counselor to carry out prescriptive recommendations in the classroom, and for the children to stay longer in the DDC.

GENERAL DISCUSSION

As the follow-up indicated, many teachers took little or no advantage of the findings and recommendations of the DDC. In some instances the recommendations were not useful. In others, the teachers did not want, or know how, to implement new teaching materials and strategies. However, our experience indicated more fundamental problems in the school and the center, problems which the DDC exposed but could not solve.

To carry out the suggested prescription, a teacher would have to make fundamental changes in her program. Most classrooms are organized around the "average child" myth. The curriculum is determined by some notions of what a child should know at a given age. Children who do not "test at grade level," or whose behavior does not conform to that which the teacher can demand of the majority of students, are seen as "aberrant" in relation to the average. Very few classrooms are organized around a diversified, individualized instructional scheme which makes it acceptable and profitable for every child to be operating at his own optimal level and speed.

There are, of course, children in many classrooms who are so disturbed that they are in need of clinical services beyond the educator's purview; or whose learning disabilities are so great that they require very special kinds of instruction. There are many more children who are labeled "aberrant" only because they do not come close enough to some myth of average, and therefore fail in classrooms which are organized around the myth. In a classroom in which reading instruction is geared to three homogeneous groups (slow, fast, and average), an individualized instructional program for one child, prescribed by the DDC, did not fit. In effect, our carefully designed program for a client required a major reorganization in the teacher's thinking and planning. What the DDC envisioned as help for a teacher around a specific child's needs was in reality a challenge to the teacher's basic concepts of educational planning. It is significant, of course, that the special class teachers were more successful in carrying out recommendations; they have smaller classes and are trained to provide individual instruction.

A related problem exposed by the DDC concerns the school's commitment to educate problem children. School systems operate an extensive network of special classrooms and other services through which they maintain problem children in school. However, there are limits of tolerance, frequently shifting and ambiguous, for each component of the network. When these limits are exceeded, the school reverses the process and the maintenance mechanism becomes an extrusion mechanism. This process can serve to relieve school personnel of their guilt feelings of failure and remove their responsibility for a child.

When a clinic automatically accepts school referrals and proceeds to apply a diagnosis and prescribe treatment, it confirms the belief of school personnel that the child cannot be served in the educational mainstream. This implies that some other group or institution must do something to bring the child's behavior into the "average" range before he can be educated. The careful, thoughtful, and rational referral of a child from a school to the mental health system can represent a useful and necessary intervention. In many instances the extrusion of a child from school into a clinic is a means the school uses to get rid of its failures.

An intervention such as the DDC runs counter to the extrusion process and thereby identifies those children who should not be caught up in it. When the psychoeducational prescription from the DDC clearly demonstrated materials and strategies which could be invoked in the classroom, it demanded further responsibility of the school. If the original motive for the referral had been to get rid of the child, the prescription could not be accepted.

This had been anticipated to some extent, and was reflected in the inclusion of the liaison counselor. Changes in that role which detracted from follow-up and classroom support were crucial. In fact, it would probably be necessary to increase the amount of attention given to inservice training of teachers in the use of unfamiliar techniques and materials. Perhaps programs such as the DDC can only be productive in relation to schools in which fundamental planned changes in philosophy and operation are directed at greater individualization of curriculum for all children. In particular, there must be a commitment toward a wider definition of "normal" and a more diversified, individualized educational program.

The DDC also exposed some problems in the center's philosophy and activities. Somewhat surprisingly, some clinical staff found it difficult, if not unnecessary, to relate their efforts with a client (and his family) to the work of the DDC. Some therapists tended to separate themselves from the client once he had been admitted to the DDC. Some failed to use the DDC staff for appropriate children on their caseload. In other cases, the necessity of collaborating with DDC staff was seen as a nuisance, just an additional complication in case planning and management. Since the center's philosophy of treatment was explicitly based on multidisciplinary, collaborative efforts, the DDC demonstrated the problems, and lack of consensus involved in that commitment.

The Children and Family Unit had also based its program on a determination to avoid programmatic divisions between mentally ill and mentally retarded children. There was some specialization of Mental Health and Mental Retardation counselors in the assignment of case responsibilities, but most staff were available to both MH and MR clients. In a large number of cases, we felt the child's IQ to be an unreliable or insignificant factor in case planning. Applying this principle to the DDC produced an uneasy arrangement which broke into conflict at points, exacerbated because most of the staffing funds for the DDC came from MR funding sources, space and equipment from MH funds. A compromise led to separate grouping of children according to primary diagnosis. The same core staff worked with all the children in the DDC.

A more fundamental issue affected those staff members who were uneasy about the place of educational activities in the basic functioning of the center. It had been assumed that the definitions of diagnosis and therapy under which the Children and Family Unit operated were broad, and could include any activity which increased our understanding of a child's needs and our ability to enhance his coping and skills. (The conceptual basis for this practice is discussed in detail in Chapter 3.) Many therapists had involved themselves in their individual casework in the child's learning problems; we had operated a tutoring program for some clients, using local high school students; we had employed an educational psychologist to broaden our evaluation; we were working directly in schools with resource rooms and remedial kinds of programs (see Chapter 5). But the creation of a room that looked somewhat like a classroom was in the judgement of some staff and administrators outside the Children and Family Unit too definitive a step into the realm of education. For them this was not the explicit business of a mental health center. For them the only legitimate activities of a mental health center were the diagnosis and treatment of those persons with mental illness. Positive intervention programs in the forms described in other chapters of this book were tolerated since they did not take place on the turf of the mental health center, but occurred in schools, welfare department, etc.

Placing the DDC in the mental health center building and stressing its educational philosophy and function was applying the "fox in the chicken coop" principle to the mental health center itself. In retrospect we believe that the kind of staff preparation and support seen as necessary to make the DDC prescriptions useful to school personnel should also be directed at center staff and administrators.

We have the following reminders to ourselves, should we ever begin another program like the DDC:

1. We would develop a method for assessing the capacity of each referring school to carry out changes in instruction and management for individual children.
2. We would carefully analyze the reasons for succeeding or failing with individual children as a basis for identifying the best candidates for the DDC.
3. We would adhere to the principle that people are more important than organizational design in linking two systems. In addition to being viewed as competent by school and clinic staff, the personnel of the DDC should work with both groups. In order to do this more effec-

tively we would combine the roles of liaison counselor and DDC teacher in one person.

4. As a condition for accepting and keeping a child in the DDC we would require that the clinic therapist and regular school teacher remain in contact with the child while he is in the DDC.

5. In order to maintain a program like the DDC, it is necessary that the administrators of school and clinic maintain close communication and assume the task of preparing and educating their respective staffs for the function of the DDC.

REFERENCES

1. Hobbs, N: Mental health's third revolution. Amer. J. Orthopsychiat. 34:822–833.

2. Valett RE: Programming Learning Disabilities. Palo Alto, California, Fearon, 1969.

3. Valett RE: The Remediation of Learning Disabilities: A Handbook of Psychoeducational Resource Programs. Belmont, California, Fearon, 1967.

4. Kirk S, Kirk W: Psycholinguistic Learning Disabilities—Diagnosis and Remediation. Urbana, Univ. Illinois Press, 1972.

5. Long NJ, Morse WC, Newman RG: Conflict in the Classroom: The Education of Children with Problems. Belmont, California, Wadsworth, 1971.

7

Consultation to a Department of Public Welfare

HIGH RISK AND LOW STATUS

One of the important criteria used in determining priorities for mental health intervention is the concept of high risk. High-risk children are those who have a greater chance of maladaptation, with the implied consequence that such maladaptation will lead to disease or disturbance in essential biopsychosocial functions. Various reports, statistical and anecdotal, have demonstrated that some children who are separated from their natural parents and placed in foster homes or group living situations frequently through public or private child welfare agencies are part of a high-risk group.[1-3] The essential condition common to these children is the experience of a significant disruption in their relationship with parents or other primary caretakers. The final act in this process when they become "children in placement" is frequently the end-result of a pattern of experiences which reflect the failure of the social bonding process.[4] Socioeconomic and psychosocial factors affecting the parents, family, and children lead to social disruption and inability or unwillingness of the parent to function effectively in his or her caregiving role. Coupled with this fundamental experience is some type of public behavior—perhaps over a period of many years—that brings the parents' distress, disturbance, and incapacity to such a level of awareness that the legal process of society intervenes and the child and parent are separated.

The work of Janice Porter Gump was essential in the theoretical and practical aspects of this program.

We know that there are many more parents whose behavior is just as inadequate as those whose children are taken from them and placed. There are parents whose failure in the parental role is just as tragic, but who never come to public attention and whose children are never placed. Which group of children are at higher risk is an important but unanswered empirical question. The necessary condition for such high risk is certainly a failure in parent-child bonding accompanying parental incapacity. The sufficient condition for placement is exposure of this behavior to the public, with subsequent intervention by the authorities. Consequently, poor parents are much more subject to having their children placed. The poor are more vulnerable to intrusion and manipulation by public authorities.

For some children, placement results in the promotion of healthy growth and development through the medium of a foster family or group living situation. The foster family provides many of the significant and crucial biological and psychosocial needs in the context of mutually satisfying relationships that the original family was unable to provide. However, some children who are placed are not as fortunate. Some are at a distinct risk for the development of subsequent severe psychological disturbances. Such an outcome may be the result of damage sustained in the original home situation or may arise from repeated failures in the placement process itself. Children whose emotional, cognitive, and social development seems most at-risk are those who are subject to repeated placements in a succession of foster homes or group living situations. This particular group of children are unable to experience the continuity of an enduring relationship with significant adults which replaces and substitutes for the original parent-child relationship. The need for such a relatively permanent relationship is one of the most singularly crucial substrates for healthy growth and development of children. Large numbers of placed children are a judgement against society and a perennial reminder of the unfilled task of that society. These children represent a challenge to the entire spectrum of human services. The way in which our country has dealt with these children and their natural parents is living proof of existing antichild and antipoor attitudes and behaviors.

Departments of welfare and their workers have been assigned one of the "dirty work" jobs of society akin to police work, garbage collection, work in correctional institutions, and state hospitals.[5,6] Because it is a "dirty work" job, the majority of the citizens and their elected representatives give it little thought so that the social and economic resources allocated to carry out this job are totally inadequate. The public gives little attention to the task of welfare except when it thinks the job is costing too much. In addition, the job itself has little status in the eyes of the delegating community. The problem of children in placement is low on the priority list of public concern or action. Children in placement are treated as second-class citizens. That these children are a public responsibility could in theory assure them of first-class treatment. Welfare, like other governmental or public functions, is of low status compared with occupations in the private sector. Ironically, the society wishes its public welfare workers to perform certain necessary tasks, but it holds the workers, their jobs, and their clients in low esteem. The public employee who tries to help children in placement is perceived as less valuable than the private employee who helps put men on the moon.

The above preamble sets the scene for the description of a consulting effort different from those described in the previous chapters. In this instance, the request came from an agency as overburdened as the school system, the Department of Public Welfare. The director of the Department of Public Welfare of the County of Philadelphia approached the director of the Temple Community Mental Health Center in the fall of 1966. The department had been awarded a grant from a private foundation to provide mental health services to those children for whom the department was responsible. The director of DPW, a veteran social worker and administrator, had as her first priority obtaining psychiatric consultative services for her social work staff. As a second priority, she wanted to provide direct services for those children most in need. At this time, only a few of the catchment areas in the city were being served by active community mental health centers. Psychiatric services for poor children were scarce and more available to those who could afford to pay. As the consultants from the Children and Family Unit became familiar with the staff and administration of the Department of Public Welfare, we also became aware of the long history of repeated attempts on the part of the department to obtain adequate services for children in placement. More often than not, these services were not obtained. More often than not, there were marked difficulties in communication and cooperative working relationships between the department and mental health clinics and agencies. More often than not, it was our impression that the mental health agencies, along with other agencies in the community, helped maintain and reinforce second-class status of department of welfare clients, in the way in which these mental health agencies dealt with both the staff of the department and their clients.

RESPONSE MODEL: YES AND NO

The consultation program we are about to describe is an example of the response model (see Chap. 5) but with a different twist. The initial contract and tentative agreement to explore the possibility of a consultation program took place with the head of the Department of Public Welfare, the director of the Temple Community Mental Health Center, and the head of its Consultation and Education Unit. Neither of the persons representing the community mental health center were to be the ones to carry out the actual consultation program. The consultation program was effected by the Director of the Children and Family Unit and a psychologist in the unit (Janice P. Gump, Ph.D.). This is a situation which occurs frequently in the beginning of a consultation effort. The boss tentatively agrees that his agency will carry out a consultation program and then passes the responsibility for planning and execution down the line to other staff. One major question needs to be asked: what are the terms of the initial tentative agreement? If it means, as it did in our case, that staff responsible for ongoing negotiations about the program could decide in the last instance not to carry out the consultation program for justifiable reasons, then the initial discussions are truly tentative in nature. If, on the other hand, the "tentative agreement" made by the mental health center director binds and commits his agency and the staff who will carry out the consultation to the development of a program, then the negotiations carried out by the consulting staff are of a much different nature. Their job then is to negotiate the best possible consulting arrangement, but they do not have the privilege of deciding after some period of discussions with the consultee agency that such a program should not be effected. It is very important that the persons who do consulting negotiations and the executing of the program be clear with their own administration about the nature and terms of the original discussion if the consulting group was not privy to these discussions.

This highlights an issue that we refer to as the "yes and no" function. When the boss says "Explore the possibilities of developing a program with this or that agency," is he really saying, "Get yourself in gear and consult to them?" or is he, in fact, saying, "Explore, look it over, and then decide." Is he saying "yes" for you or do you still retain the power to say "no"? (There is a fuller discussion of the notion of the "yes and no" function as it relates to organizational roles in Chapter 11.) In the first instance, the boss has exercised the definitive "yes" function. The staff members who are to consult have the task of negotiating the most reasonable program possible within the usual limits of time, personnel, money, and the interaction between the expectations of the requesting agency and the capabilities of the consulting group. In this situation, the consultant must be very clear with his own boss about the time, staff, and other services, that can be used in developing a program. The consultant needs to know from his boss whether this is an add-on program that the mental health center is committed to no matter how hard it squeezes available resources, or whether this is a program that takes priority over some other program and thus allows for a shifting of the available resources. Resources of time and people are always overextended. The issue is whether they will be more overextended by simply getting more work out of everybody or whether a trade-off is possible in that taking on X allows us to not do or decrease doing Y. The consultant who works for a mental health center, or who is not simply a solo practitioner, must have a clear notion from his own boss of the risks, benefits, politics, and finances which make his boss decide to take on a particular program.

A good rule is: when a boss voluntarily agrees to provide service to another group or agency when this particular service is not mandated by law, there are undoubtedly political considerations, financial considerations, and personal considerations, or all three involved in that decision. With the Temple Mental Health Center, the political considerations were those of establishing a presence, a reputation, a model community mental health center in Philadelphia, and hopefully for the country. The financial considerations were less prominent but important since the center was reimbursed through the foundation grant for the time the consultants spent working with the agency. Nevertheless, the consultant group in the Children and Family Unit had real autonomy and retained a "yes-no" function. We could have chosen not to become involved in the consultation program. Each year at the contract renewal time, we knew that we could have chosen not to renegotiate or reenter the program with the agency if we felt that it was not productive or if we felt that some other demands relating to the goals of the Children and Family Unit were more important.

THE CONTRACT: HOW WILL WE DO WHAT TO WHOM AND WHY?

Ormsby[7] and Bernard[8] have provided general descriptions of consultation to social agencies. Rosenthal and Sullivan[9] present a detailed description of a case-centered consultation project carried out with the Illinois Department of Public Welfare in the midfifties. Although we began with a case consultation model, we built in certain characteristics that allowed for elaboration and development through other consultative activities. By the end of 4 years, a consultation structure had evolved which could serve as a model for a consulting program, not only to departments of public welfare but also to similar agencies providing human services. From the beginning, the consultants had the goal of developing such a model as part of the explicit negotiation with the director of the public welfare agency.

The beginnings of the development of the program centered on the director and her administrative cabinet. This cabinet was composed of assistant director and section chiefs of the various major units; direct service, intake and protective services, purchase of care, and adoptive services. At the outset, the consultant suggested and the welfare administrators agreed that review and planning sessions would constitute a central feature of our consultation program. The review and planning group included the consultants, the director of the agency, and her administrative cabinet. Initially, the most important use of such a meeting was that of staff preparation. Joint meetings were held between the consultants and different levels of agency personnel: administration, supervisors, and caseworkers to facilitate a clear communication to as much of the staff as possible about what the consultants intended to do. Equally important, these meetings established a face-to-face relationship between consultants and their future consultees. The initial phase of contract negotiation is crucial and is discussed in several other chapters in this book. The next phase of consultation development, that of establishing face-to-face relationships with the consultee group warrants a good deal of time and effort. Adequate attention paid to this phase will reap an equally high reward throughout the consultation program.

REVIEW AND PLANNING FUNCTION

Review and planning meetings served as a vehicle for ongoing examination and implementation of the entire program. Such a regularly recurring meeting provides an opportunity for dealing with anxieties and concerns about mental health, in general, and in the real and fantasied effects that the consultant may have on the agency and its staff. These meetings provide a definitively scheduled time to deal with complaints and the problems with the consulting program as they arise from any level within the agency. Reciprocally, the complaints and problems of consultants are aired to the agency administrators. For example, one of the problems that arose in the beginning of the program and recurred throughout the 4 years was the slowness in readying cases for presentation, or at times, a total lack of case consultation requests. Such occasions provided the consultants and the administrative cabinet an opportunity to examine what this behavior might mean. For instance, it may mean that the staff was so overwhelmed with their ordinary duties and case responsibilities that they did not have time to develop a case for presentation. Or, alternatively, it might mean that the supervisors were not inquiring of staff whether or not there were problem cases around for which they wanted help. Alternatively, it might occur at a time of high staff turnover with old workers leaving and new workers coming in to the agency. These new workers may not have been oriented to the possibility of mental health consultation for their clients. In addition, for new workers, the anxiety of being new to their jobs made consultation rather low on their priority list.

Planning and review sessions provided an opportunity to look at what had been going on in previous months and an opportunity to adjust and modify the program. A pertinent example: after the first 3 months suggestions were made by the agency to add topical discussions around certain general kinds of issues relating to mental health, that is, the runaway child. Such problems faced many workers in their day-to-day work. The supervisory and administrative staff of the agency wanted to have their workers informed as to how to interpret this behavior and, more important, how to be helpful both to the child and the foster family.

Another important and ongoing discussion that arose early and provided a recurring leitmotif, concerned role boundaries and role overlap. A variety of questions arose, but they could be reduced to crucial ones about role functions summarized in the following way. What is a psychiatric or mental health problem? What is a casework problem? How do the two overlap or intermingle, and how are they distinct? The agency was uncomfortable in that it might be presenting cases which "weren't sick enough" or "weren't serious enough," and which might be construed by the consultants as indicating that the agency had not done its casework job. The agency administrators felt it might appear that mental health consultants were being asked to comment on casework problems rather than on "mental health problems." The consultants, on the other hand, were worried about being overwhelmed with a number of severely disturbed children for whom they could not provide or find adequate services. Initially, the planning and review sessions allowed the consultants the opportunity to offer reassurance to the administrators and through them to the staff concerning this issue. We defined our view of mental health as broad rather than narrow, focusing on psychosocial functioning and adaptation rather than on narrow categories of illness or symptom-related behaviors. We encouraged any caseworker who was uncomfortable about a child to consider this child as a possible candidate for consultation and to proceed to approach her supervisor for further exploration. We promoted a more generic view of the helping process rather than trying to split hairs over what was casework territory and what was mental health territory. A final use of the planning and review session provided an opportunity to move beyond case consultation and into the area of administrative and program consultation.

STAFF PREPARATION

As mentioned above, the planning and review session developed a phasing-in period for the consultants to get to know the work and organization of the agency. During this period, the consultants reviewed some of the written material which had defined the mission and role of the agency and its relation to other agencies within the city government structure. In addition, the consultants read the yearly reports of the director and the commissioner of public welfare which summarized the functions and operations of the department on an annual basis. We requested and received permission to review a number of case records picked at random to become more informed about the problems of children and the agency.

We established a number of staff preparation meetings moving from the administrative to supervisory and on to line staff levels. These meetings allowed for an explanation of the nature of the consultation program and questions and prospective problems could be raised. The meetings also offered an opportunity for staff to suggest ways in which the program might be more practically useful to them and thus helped shape the program before it became operative. Such meetings also attended to the important but covert issues that can be epitomized in the following questions: Who are you? What are you doing here? Who do you work for? What are you going to offer me? What are you going to expect of me? These questions are basic and form the matrix of the initial stages of all human relationships. They are generally raised in and camouflaged in oblique ways. It is important for consultants to be able to identify the basic nature of these questions, and to respond to them beneath the camouflage as directly and unthreateningly as possible. At the more explicit level there are questions such as: Are those consultants going to tell us what is wrong with us? Are they going to psych us? Are they really going to be of any help to me with my kids or are they merely going to give me a lot of jargon and suggestions that are of little practical help?

We as consultants had our own concerns which we also expressed at times obliquely; but as we became more comfortable, we were able to express more directly. Is the agency going to expect the impossible? Are they going to ask us to pull rabbits out of hats? Are we supposed to be able to treat all these children they refer to us for consultation? When the agency is unable to place a difficult child, will this child suddenly become a mental health or psychiatric emergency, and will we be required to find a hospital or residential setting for him? Are caseworkers getting in over their heads and trying to be therapists when they have neither the time nor perhaps training and experience to adequately function in this role?

Each side's questions were raised early but could not be worked out merely by words. It requires time and working together around common concerns and tasks for "the answers" to some of these questions to become clear. For some questions, it requires time for all parties to know that significant and definitive answers do not exist. Some problems are always problems, some problems are not soluble; they are just constantly reworked and are endured. Such problems include the lack of staff, lack of sufficient time for any one case, lack of adequate referral sources. However, the mutual support, trust, and help the consultants and counsultees provided for each other made some problems easier to endure and confront.

CASE CONSULTATION: FORMAT

The centerpiece of the consultation involved group meetings with staff in which one or two children or families were discussed. With the administrative cabinet and with the larger group of 30 supervisors, we established a preparation procedure for the consultation sessions.

1. The caseworker determined with her supervisor which case or cases presented the most serious concerns. The initial concern could begin with a supervisor who then brought it to the attention of the responsible caseworker.
2. The caseworker wrote up a summary of the case following a protocol the consultants had prepared. According to the protocol, the worker first spelled out in some detail specific questions and concerns she had regarding the case and to which she wished the consultants to respond. She listed the specific behaviors, events, or conditions that gave rise to her questions. A brief summary of the child's history, with special emphasis on the placement history and developmental progress was noted. Instances of specific strengths of the child as well as evidence of maladaptation to major environments, foster homelife, school, and peers were included. The overall written material averaged one and a half to two typewritten pages.

The consultants were ambivalent at first about requiring such a protocol, fearing it would discourage consultation requests. As a group, welfare workers are overwhelmed with paper work and record keeping. As in hospitals and schools, a case can be made that much of the staff time is involved in "treating the record," not the client. However, there is an important and necessary function of such voluminous records in welfare departments. For many children, especially those experiencing multiple placements, the record contains their life thread. Successive foster parents may know only a smattering of the child's previous life. They certainly do not know it with the intimacy and immediacy they would if they had experienced this life with the child. Social worker turnover is high and thus for many children, the agency records are truly the archives of their lives.

The consultants were encouraged and supported in the expectation of the written protocol by the director and her assistants. All felt it would make consultation sessions more focused and productive. The director of Inservice Training, a former dean of a school of social work, also supported the procedure, feeling it would be a useful learning experience for the workers. Their advice proved to be correct. In addition, the act of writing up the protocol, especially the initial expectation of specifying the question or issues for the consultant, initiated a self-help process for the worker. Since self-help is always a crucial aspect of consultation and therapeutic endeavors, the write-up provided a vehicle for the initial phase of the consultation, promoting the initiative of the worker as a priority from the beginning.

The children selected by the workers for consultative help were, except a few, exhibiting behaviors which severely stressed either the foster parents directly or indirectly through the child's behaviors at school. This stress was, in turn, experienced by the department. The child was presenting a threat either to his placement (if he continues these behaviors, the foster parents will demand his removal) or a threat to the agency's resources—(dare we risk another foster home on this boy when he has had trouble in so many?) Basically, the child's behavior presented a threat to his own present and future adaptation because of the negative reactions they produced in those around him. Such were the fundamental reasons underlying the request for consultative help, even though the explicit reasons were very often differently stated. Initially, then, the consultants dealt with the central issue of restating or reformulating the reason for consultation. This restatement was not simply a rephrasing; it required that everyone begin to look at the case or the problem in a different conceptual framework. The conceptual schema found useful was that of the notion of social system. The consultants viewed the child not as an isolated psychiatric problem to be solved, but rather as one link of an interrelated network comprised of foster family, child, school, and agency. Each of these entities and their interrelationships had to be examined if resolution of the presenting problem were to be approached. This is not to say that the consultants felt it unimportant to examine specific psychological issues such as, what is the meaning of the child's sexual acting out? Or, could this child's enuresis be related to neurological impairment? We attempted to answer such questions both with reference to the specific case as well as in more general terms. We believed that consultation is an educative process, not only around specific case-related issues but also involving more contextual issues not as easily identified by the consultee because he is embedded in the process and the system itself.

PROFILES: CHILD

What are the "typical" kinds of problems presented for case consultation? First, in line with our notion of examining the system, we present an abstract and acknowledgedly stereotypic profile of a child presented for consultation. Note that often there is one caseworker responsible for the child and another for the foster parents who are caring for the child. Often there might be more than one caseworker responsible for different children placed in the same home depending on time and circumstance of placement. Thus, the system is very complex and coordination of care was often difficult to achieve. What we present here in the way of profiles are composites and in no way express the complex individual variations among children, foster parents, and workers.

In the majority of cases, the child presented for consultation was a boy. He was black, in the preadolescent age range, 10 or 11 years old. More often than not, he had been separated from his family since his preschool years. He frequently had more than one foster home placement, including an initial "temporary" placement that could have lasted up to 2 years. (Ideally, temporary placement lasts approximately 3 months so the child can be adequately evaluated and a suitable foster home selected for him. Frequently, this ideal was not met because of the chronic shortage of foster homes available for long-term placement.) The child is often one to two grades below expected educational attainment. He shares this situation with many poor urban children whether they live with their natural or foster families. The problem behavior he presents is typical of the kinds of problems of all children who become of concern to those around them: disruptive behavior in class, defiance at home, lying, stealing, occasional delinquent acts, withdrawal and negativism, running away, and underachievement. Sexual disturbances were rare as a primary complaint. Many of these children have a characteristic disturbance in interpersonal relationships that goes back to the original difficulty they experienced in some of the early social bonding with parents. Often, subsequent substitutive relationships were also broken, contributing to the major difficulty that many of these children had in establishing mutually satisfactory interpersonal relationships with adults and peers. Out of these experiences developed a psychosocial set that included the expectation of being disappointed, a certain feeling of futility and fatalism, and clinical symptoms of overt or masked depression. Some children adopted as protection a superficial but effective ability to ingratiate themselves and relate to adults easily, but rather shallowly. This again was a reflection of their need to cope with repeated changes in significant relationships. The more successful of the children found a way of learning to perceive and adapt to adult expectations, giving just as much as necessary to maintain themselves in an environment that could be changed tomorrow for reasons they little understood and for which they felt responsible.

PROFILE: FOSTER PARENTS

The foster parents were likewise a heterogeneous group, predominantly black, since the highest proportion of poor children at-risk to go into placement were black. An oversimplified profile reveals that the foster parents were over 40, father a skilled workman, and the mother a housewife most of her life. Together, they had raised several children of their own, many of whom were grown and married. A notable percentage had been foster children themselves. Frequently, some of the couple's natural children were still living in the house but were usually in the mid or late teens. Foster parents tended to be people with a strong sense of personal and social tradition. They were church goers, had a highly ingrained sense of right and wrong, and of what was expected and appropriate behavior for children. They were not particularly psychologically minded people, nor were they consumers of much of the vast psychologically oriented literature regarding child rearing, marriage, and family life. They believed in firm, but fair discipline. They were not adverse to spanking when they felt it was indicated, even though this was a strict taboo of the agency. They were sensitive to and aware of the privations and traumas that children had experienced before being placed with them. At times, they saw themselves involved in a making-up sort or relationship or being a good parent for the child who had previously only experienced "bad parents." These foster parents expected much of the children and they expected even more of themselves. They often persisted with children in spite of significant behavior difficulties not with just one but with several of the children in their care. Many of them wanted to hang on longer than they could or should. They did not like to fail in anything. The women, in particular, whose major role identity was tied up in motherhood, had a great investment in succeeding with the children.

In short, these foster parents were admirable upholders of the major traditional American values. They believed that they had something to offer children that could help them grow and develop into useful citizens and adults. They did not make the common mistake of many of the so-called psychologically sophisticated professionals in seeing these children as total victims of forces beyond their control. Such a view which is frequently fomented by psychological theory and practice not only explains behavior, but runs the risk of removing from the child the opportunity and expectation of developing reasonable responsibility for his behavior and taking charge of his destiny. Frequently, the foster parents were responsible for raising several children from different natural families, oftentimes very close in age and coming into placement at rather different times. Repeatedly, the consultants were impressed with the almost overwhelming magnitude of the task many of these foster parents faced. They persisted with dedication, devotion, sacrifice, and little or no promise of reward except what was brought about by living up to their own ideals and goals. These men and women are some of the unsung heroes and heroines of society, doing the "dirty work," sharing the status of the children and caseworkers, receiving little from society in terms of recognition, esteem, or money for their efforts.

PROFILE: CASEWORKERS

Caseworkers in the department were on the average a good deal younger than the foster parents with whom they related. The average caseworker was a woman in her midtwenties, though in the latter 1960s, an increasing number of young men came into the department. Some of the caseworkers were trained social workers at a masters level, others were not. Those who were untrained had college degrees. There were more white than black caseworkers, although supervisory staff were in the majority black. Their socioeconomic and educational levels were higher than those of the foster parents or children they served. In general, the caseworker focused on the needs of children and construed her role as helping effect the fulfillment of these needs through the aegis of the foster parents. Sociopolitically, the views of the caseworkers tended to be more liberal than those of the foster parents. In contrast to the common sense, traditional approach to childrearing, caseworkers were more imbued with psychological mindedness and psychological information. Much of this was theoretical knowledge, for they were for the most part unmarried and had never borne or raised children. Some of them had previous experience in day camps, babysitting, and as siblings in their own families. However, it is not an overstatement to say that, in general, caseworkers were long on theory and short on practice with regard to children. In turn, the foster parents' practical experience was extensive, but frequently they were limited in their overall conception of the needs of childhood, particularly in a psychological and emotional area. Clashes between worker and parents, when they occurred, were mainly caused by a difference in perspective with regard to children. Given the basic goodwill and the dedication of both foster parents and caseworkers each to their own role and task, fairly effective compromises were worked out when conflicts arose.

In the case consultation sessions, the consultants highlighted these differences. The social system framework helped the caseworker take some distance in seeing these issues not as related so much to individual personal dynamics, right or wrong attitudes, or practices toward child-rearing, but as differences that resulted from a multiplicity of factors related to age, experience, socioeconomic class, and education. These factors strongly influenced the particular way a social worker or foster parent each viewed his or her role in relationship to the children, to the agency, and to each other.

CASE CONSULTATION: PROCESS

Specifically, we carried out our consultation as follows. Having reviewed the protocol submitted to us prior to the consultation, we met at a prearranged scheduled place and time with a small group, administratively designated as the unit, which consisted of four to eight social workers under the direction of the supervisor. Since all had been privy to the protocol material prior to the meeting, we were able to begin with substantive issues. If there had been some delay between the date of the submission of the protocol and the date of consultation, we asked the worker to review the intervening events.

The psychiatrist and psychologist functioned as a team in the first 2 years of the program. The advantages of team consultation are several. We divided our roles so that one of us agreed to be in charge of the consultation for that day or session. He or she then orchestrated the presentation and generally directed the overall focus of the meeting. Prior to the meeting, the consultants had met and discussed their opinions of the protocol, exchanged ideas and had an overall notion of the approach they would take or the issues they would highlight. Just as in cotherapy, a coconsultant arrangement can be very useful when one supplements the other in a number of ways. When one consultant is actively eliciting questions, responding to comments, or promoting group interaction, the coconsultant can be observing how the group is responding, the degree of participation of various members, and whether or not the approach of the consultant is clear. Further, the coconsultant who is less active has a better opportunity to pick up some of the affective tone in the interaction between the consultant and consultees and can intervene as he or she sees necessary. Another very useful advantage of coconsultancy is that the consultants can take different points of view, thus encouraging through their own modeling behavior the notion that there is not just one way to look at a particular phenomena or only one way to deal with it.

Since the coconsultants each represented different mental health disciplines which, at times, have status problems and territorial disputes, it was an advantage for the consultees to be able to see a psychiatrist and psychologist working together, alternating roles of dominance and leadership, and dealing essentially with each other as colleagues who respected each other's professional skills and personal contributions. We also could acknowledge to each other and with the consultees our own limitations, which derived from our particular training and professional background or from the nature of the case itself which did not admit any "solutions."

Our behavior in consultation was active, asking questions, and in general taking charge of the focus and direction of the consultation fairly explicitly. We promoted a free exchange of ideas and opinions and feelings among the consultees. We wanted to use this vehicle as a model for the consultees to have the various social workers and supervisors listen to each other, to learn from each other's experience, and to recognize that they have much to offer each other about their particular problems with difficult cases. We did not eschew or avoid the role of experts who were willing to provide information, take a definitive stand, or at times be authoritative. However, we balanced these behaviors by strongly promoting the mutual support of the group, not only emotionally but particularly in terms of experience sharing. We promoted the kind of interaction in which one worker would say to another, "You know, when I had a problem like that with a child, these were some of the things I tried." The adressee would respond saying, "Well, how did you find out about this?" Or, "I tried that and it did not work so well because . . ."

We knew that caseworkers were overburdened with large numbers of cases and administrative responsibilities. They frequently operated alone in the field, visiting the homes, involved in a hectic daily pace. They needed the opportunity to share with each other not only their difficulties in order to obtain effective emotional release and support but an opportunity to come to know that each had something to offer the other about the tasks at hand.

The consultants themselves respected the skills and experience of the workers and their ingenuity with overwhelming problems. By making explicit this interest and respect and by querying the workers about how they solved a particular problem or approached a particularly difficult foster parent, the consultants were able to elicit from the various workers what they did and how they did it. At times, this engendered a healthy difference of opinion and disagreement. At other times, it was clear that the jockeying for position with relation to supervisors took place when one worker tried to appear better or more acceptable or more knowledgeable than another. These were facets of the process the consultants had to face and deal with on the spot, recognizing the personal, professional, administrative, and status issues involved when workers and supervisors are in the same group.

PURPOSES OF CONSULTATION

The case consultation sessions served several purposes. They provided a fairly expeditious way of bringing to the attention of the consultant those children for whom there was concern regarding a possibility of serious mental disturbance. The consultation in these situations focused on whether there was a need for further diagnostic services or treatment services, the nature of the mental disturbance involved, and the possible intrapsychic, intrafamilial, and psychosocial dynamics. When indicated either by residence in the Temple Community Mental Health catchment area or by lack of available service in the area in which the child resided, diagnostic or treatment services or both were provided by the Temple Community Mental Health Center Children and Family Unit. Thus, the consultants in some cases had both a consultative and a direct service relationship to some of the children and foster families.

In other instances, the consultation was intended to help the worker identify and clarify the particular needs of a given child in terms of placement, schooling, and relationship to foster or natural family, or both. In these instances, understanding and planning a course of action or alternative courses of action were the prime issues in consultation.

Emergency situations in which very complicated, intrapsychic, intrafamilial, and social reality factors combined with a crisis event caused the worker or supervisor to use whatever resources were available to them including mental health consultation. Often in such circumstances because of slow bureaucratic procedures, the child was unable to get the emergency services he needed. At times, the consultants were helpful in using their "union card" to prevail on a mental health or hospital facility to provide emergency care for this child. (Parenthetically, one should note that one of the standard responses in most hospital emergency rooms, including those of pediatric hospitals to any kind of disturbed child is literally, "Get him out of here." These are the same emergency rooms with highly skilled staff who can deal with a physically traumatized child, the convulsing child, the burned child, or the child in severe status asthmaticus. But the disturbed or disturbing child finds no place in the hospital emergency room. This is clearly a concrete point at which the medical model of "mental illness" and the response system for the disturbance are incongruent and incompatible. If such children are mentally ill, they are the primary responsibility of the medical community. Hospital emergency rooms, particularly pediatric emergency rooms, have absolutely no right to refuse whatever treatment is needed for these children.)

Other consultations were focused on the worker's relationship with the child and the foster family. The worker's feeling and responses were aired as these related to her role. Consultants maintained a careful boundary line between the role behaviors and difficulties versus the intrapsychic and personal problems that the worker might have. When we felt that the worker or the group was intruding too much into the personal and intrapsychic area of the worker's personality, we reshifted the focus to concentrate on role and work behaviors. In doing this, we clearly recognized that certain role behaviors are affected by intrapsychic dynamics and difficulties. The strategy in this case is one of focus and emphasis rather than the refusal to recognize a close relationship between personal issues and role behaviors. We strongly believed that the focus on role was more appropriate and effective for a consultation relationship, particularly in a group. Focus on personal issues could be appropriate in the supervisory relationship or possibly in a one-to-one consulting situation when consultant and consultee have established a trusting and open relationship and made such discussion an explicit part of their working contract.

Cases were presented that were examples of multiple or agency or multiple worker involvement. A common situation was one in which a worker was terminating with a family or child and another worker or entire unit was initiating the care or responsibility for the child or family. In these instances, the consultants attempted to facilitate transitions, clarify the nature of separations and beginnings, and make explicit the feelings involved—anxiety, depression, anger, uncertainty, and loss, which touched everyone, child, foster family, and worker. Even supervisors who did not have direct contact with the child or family experienced some of the difficult feelings around such separations and transitions. The consultants promoted the relationship between the worker and supervisor in suggesting that such discussions of these feelings continue after the consultation session between worker and supervisor. We had decided that part of our role was to promote and support the administrative and structural relationships of the agency and to enhance the support mechanisms that a worker could get through his or her supervisor. Such an approach also helped reinforce this facet of the supervisor's role.

TOPICAL DISCUSSIONS

In addition to case consultation, we offered topical discussions to larger groups of staff. These dealt with issues and problems chosen by the staff and were relevant to their work. Topics included psychosis, sexually deviant behavior, parenting behavior, runaway behavior, antisocial behavior, and cognitive development and cognitive stimulation. Other topics focused on family dynamics, the battered-child syndrome, discipline and childrearing techniques, psychiatric diagnoses and treatment, and the uses of psychological testing. We kept these groups to a size of 20 or 30 so that discussion and interchange could take place. The consultant's approach was not to have all the answers, but to provide definitive and explicit information when there was knowledge and to highlight conflicting views and opinions when there was no sound scientific evidence or when various theories and approaches seemed equally useful. We again used the group process to promote interchange and sharing of information and ideas among group members so that staff as well as consultants were able to provide answers as well as questions.

STRATEGIES, TACTICS, AND THEMES

What sort of approaches and themes did the consultants use in their case consultations? We felt that the initial effort in pushing hard for workers to examine what they were really asking in seeking consultation was not only useful in the particular consultation sessions but could be carried over in the worker's everyday activities. We hoped that our questioning would promote a process of careful examination of the problems, behaviors, and questions that arose around work with a child and how these issues were bothersome to the child himself, the foster parents, the school, or to the worker and the agency. This sort of clarification took a good deal of time and occasionally a second consultation session on the same child was necessary. Consultation sessions provided an opportunity for affective release and exploration. The workers expressed concern and doubt about what they were doing, about agency policies and procedures, and about the choice of foster parents. Workers were angry at living situations in which children were placed, and they were also angry at the children who were not living up to the worker's expectations or who were inadvertently putting the workers in a dilemma by their behaviors. Anger at times extended to the children's natural parents for their acts and failures that resulted in the child's placement in the first place. Such issues should be expected in consultation and need to be faced explicitly. At the same time, it is important to know what issues to deal with and when. Consultants should not be drawn in to intraagency disputes when they revolve around personality conflicts or administrative and policy disagreements. This is the "let's you and him fight" situation.[10] Related to this Bernean game is another important and recurring theme, the one of "ain't it awful."[11] This theme frequently arises among people who are overwhelmed and feel powerless to do anything about their situation, and manifests itself as a mutually escalating chorus of complaints without any real energy directed toward problem solving.

In dealing with the issue of "let's you and him fight," consultants need to make permissible the notion that disagreements can exist between personnel in terms of their personal view of the policies and procedures of the agency. Discussion of this disagreement and an expression or difference of opinion is healthy and useful. The consultants need to point out that there ought to be and probably are channels within an agency to express disagreements with the administration and to make suggestions for alternatives. Consultants ought to stress strongly that those who complain about policy or procedures have the responsibility, if they are serious about it, to offer reasonable alternatives. These alternatives need to be construed in terms of usefulness and feasibility, and must recognize the political realities of any public agency and how these affect policy and procedures. Certainly, it is important that the consultants stand for open and free discussion among subordinates and superiors, and model for superiors the function of free discussion within reasonable bounds.

Consultants can also point out to subordinates and line workers that frequently they have a magical view of the omnipotence and power of administrators. The view is that if only the administrators wanted to change something, they could do it by fiat, by memo, or by a simple change of mind. Such oversimplified thinking must be made explicit for what it is, and replaced by a more realistic view of the limited power of administrators as well as the complexities involved in carrying out changes in policies and procedures in a cumbersome and bureaucratic society. To say this is the way things are is not to say that one should like it or think it is the best way to do things.

The other game, "Ain't it awful," should be labeled clearly for what it is—an expression of feelings of helplessness, powerlessness, and anger at those things over which people feel they have no control. The consultants can make a realistic examination of why a worker feels helpless. The next step is to identify issues in the case that the worker feels are essential to affect. The next step is to examine the alternatives a worker has and what she can do in effecting a change in a foster parent, a school, or a child. Next in problem solving is to pick among the cardinal issues the ones that appear amenable to a worker's efforts. Finally, the consultants help the worker establish a step-by-step procedure by which she can deal with those one or two issues that are important and that can be influenced. There are two processes involved: first, the empathic recognition of the feelings of helplessness and frustration, and second, the development of a task orientation so that worker can move to a position of greater competence, initiating role-appropriate and practical interventions.

The consultant found another process very important, namely, ignorance sharing. We were frequently asked to comment on the predictability of outcome of one type of foster placement over another for a particular child. Directly expressing our ignorance, we made clear as well the limits of psychiatric and psychologic knowledge concerning such predictions. We particularly supported the importance of the segment of real life that the workers experienced with the child and his family. We contrasted this with the kind of narrow "in vitro" view that a mental health worker obtains with a child or family in an office interview.

Another approach we used was that of spontaneous humor. We poked fun at ourselves, at the pedantry of mental health professionals, and at the preciousness of the respective theories involved in explaining human behavior. At times, even in very serious and difficult problems and dilemmas, we would invoke humor or workers would relate a humorous anecdote. Humor seems to be one of the major coping mechanisms of human beings. Offer has pointed out in his longitudinal study of normal adolescents that humor is frequently used as an effective coping device for adolescents in their development.[12] Stories from wartime and natural catastrophes are frequently interlaced and spiced with humorous anecdotes. We found that humor and absurdity even in the most difficult situations provides a release for feelings and also some distance and perspective on the situation as well as on the self.

The consultant frequently took a "doesn't everyone" attitude. This was used particularly when workers were responding in an overly surprised, shocked, or censorious manner toward the feelings and behaviors of the foster parents or children or even toward their own feelings and attitudes. We tried as much as possible to encourage the natural acceptance of a wide range of feelings and behaviors as being common to everyone and not a peculiarity that was visited on only the particular population that the workers encountered.

We took strong issue with the endemic "try to make up for" notion that pervades a good deal of work with psychologically or socially damaged children. We stated rather explicitly and boldly that there is no way a worker or foster parent or anyone can make up for or make up to children the devastations and failures in human relationships that they were unfortunate enough to experience. The issue we stressed constantly was that it was not reasonable to try "to make up for" but to attempt to make life from here on and from now on, reasonable and positive in terms of the kinds of experiences and relationships the children had. We pointed out to the workers that they could help the foster parents in ridding themselves of the burden of this catch-up or make-up sort of approach to children. Such an approach can, at times, lead to overindulgence of a child by the adults. As the child gets older, he can learn to use this mechanism to tyrannize and control adults by acting as though the world owed him a mother, or a better deal. The use of this psychological tactic leads to more self-defeating and disappointing relationships.

We took a modified view of the recurrent shibboleth, quite common among the mental health brotherhood, that the expression of feelings under any and all circumstances is a general mental health vitamin. Sometimes a worker elicits strong feelings of anger, disappointment, and rage from a child in a once every 2- to 3-month visit, with the naïve notion that it is somewhat therapeutic and helpful. This tactic leaves the child unprotected and vulnerable to both his own feelings and the consequences when he subsequently expresses the same strong feelings to his foster parents or his teacher. He may then find himself the object of retaliation for what those adults see as defiant behavior that they have to stamp out. We discouraged the workers from getting in too deep with some of the very painful and deep feelings of loss and hurt the children may have experienced in their lives, especially in the breakup of the early relationship with their parents. We stressed the positive and coping side of such things as denial, avoidance, and suppression of the strong feelings connected with very deep and devastating experiences over which the child had no control and for which he can do nothing *now*.

We put strong emphasis on dealing with the here and now, the life the child was leading in the present, and the people he was leading it with, the other foster children, his own siblings, and his foster parents. We stressed that feelings in those situations can be encouraged and elicited as they might serve to help the child understand himself, to come to a better acceptance of himself, and to learn a more effective way of dealing with others. We certainly wanted the workers to be sensitive and aware of their own feelings and to use them as guidelines in their relationships with the child and foster family.

In the group consultations, we repeatedly stressed the following points: first, the importance of human relationships for children's development and healthy adjustment; second, the importance of cognitive control, in other words, the importance of making sense of things. Although this is an important issue for everyone, it is particularly important for the foster child in making sense of his own life, which included his own history. Information about himself, about his past, and information that might prepare him for the future in terms of anticipatory guidance were seen as crucial activities that the worker can engage in both with the child directly and indirectly through her work with the foster parents. Thus, the child needs to be prepared for the possibility of being moved and needs to know what may happen to him and why. The worker must give him direct and honest explanations, without trying to protect either the child or herself by avoidance and deviousness. Third, we stressed the importance of competence, that is, being good at something. We said that competence is very important for all and kept asking workers to look for ways in which they could help children take advantage of their abilities, whatever they were good at in their natural life setting.[13] Competence is especially critical for these children, who, in general, must be more self-reliant and more autonomous because of the pilgrim-like existence they are forced to lead. There is as much risk for them in too much dependency as there is in no investment in others at all.

These children, more than others, are acted upon, are done to, and thus they are more likely than other children to become fatalists, to see themselves as victims without being able to initiate, but only respond. Not having the knowledge or information of why things happen to them or why and how decisions are made, these children need a large input of information and explanation so that at least they can be helped to make sense out of things, even when that sense is very painful. This is why adults often fail to give information to them, in order to protect the children and indirectly protect themselves. In the long run, however, this protection is false and is nowhere near as protective and self-arming as knowledge and information supportively given and explained.

In addition to knowledge and information, the guiding adult must be able to respect and tolerate the multiple feelings the child may experience as he tries to deal with experiences of rejection, failure, and loss. Children all have a tendency to personalize in an egocentric manner, seeing all events as revolving around their own causality. These foster children may see themselves as the cause of their parents' original decision to place them or of the subsequent replacement decisions made by one foster family after another. The children are quite likely to begin to incorporate a feeling of intrinsic badness or worthlessness. It takes all the skill that any helper can provide to help overcome and counterbalance the tremendous assault on self-esteem gathered from these repeated painful losses and separations.

Finally, we recognized and called attention to the multiple complex roles which can serve as a source of conflict and frustration for the worker. Such tasks include relating to the child, gaining information and support from the foster parents, being cast in the role of policeman to see that agency policies are being carried out, and throughout being a person who strives to be humanly responsible to the child and the parents.

ADMINISTRATIVE AND PROGRAM CONSULTATION

The planning and review sessions which were a fixed and regularly scheduled part of the consultation program provided a natural opportunity to move into programmatic and administrative consultative efforts. In fact, there is no sharp distinction between program or administrative consultation and some may use the terms interchangeably. In our view, program consultation occurs when an agency invites a consultant to help it evaluate or improve an ongoing service component or to assist in the development of a new program congruent with the agency's mission and responsibilities. Administrative consultation focuses more on the internal policies, procedures, decision making, and hierarchical relationships of the agency and the way it allocates resources of time, people, and money. In this perspective, program consultation is more concrete, specific, task-oriented, and more directly related to the service output function of an agency. Administrative consultation is more inward looking, is more concerned with "process," and more likely tends to examine the typical ways the agency is doing things in general or around specific problems and concerns. Such are the logical and theoretical distinctions. In practice, the two are often intertwined, although there is a fairly clear awareness in the consultant's as well as the consultee's mind when the consultant enters the "inner sanctum" of the administrative consultative relationship. Caplan, in his recent work on mental health consultation, and McClung and Stunden, authors of an HEW monograph on mental health consultation to children's programs, present typologies of mental health consultation and the criteria characterizing each of the different types.[14,15]

Several important opportunities for program consultation arose during our work with the Department of Public Welfare, but we will only describe two in this chapter. One example of program consultation centers on the concern the department had in developing closer ties to their foster parents as a group. This interest long antedated the arrival of the consultants to the agency. During the first year of the planning and review sessions, the director and her administrators explained some of the goals and ideas they had in promoting a more effective relationship with foster parents as a group. They wanted to increase the communication and understanding among agency staff, administration, and foster parents. They wanted to help foster parents become better informed about agency policies and procedures and to become convinced that the agency was available to them for support and help. The department officials also wanted to provide an opportunity for foster parents to give feedback to the agency about their particular experiences with children and with the agency. The consultants strongly supported and encouraged this approach. Further, we suggested some additional components of program development that might meet some of the psychological needs and interests of foster parents.

We indicated that one of the functions of small group meetings of foster parents, whether with agency staff or alone, would be to provide mutual support to each other and to share some of their experiences and expertise about caring for children in placement. This approach paralleled the model that the consultants promoted with the mutual support aspect of the case consultation meetings with groups of staff. A second and related idea was that the agency might promote a "buddy" system in which the more experienced foster parents could provide advice and support to novice foster parents through the medium of a hotline telephone or through personal acquaintanceship. If the foster parents group were to organize effectively, its officers or representatives could meet occasionally with the administrative cabinet of the agency to discuss areas of common concern, problems, and misunderstandings. In addition, the foster parent group could serve as an effective community advocacy group to inform the public at large of the needs of foster children and of the significant functions of foster parents. Finally, extending one of our basic notions of taking advantage of the expertise and experience of natural caretakers, we suggested that some carefully selected foster parents could on occasion be used in helping screen candidates who are applying to become foster parents. These veteran foster parents might be in a better position to make some judgment, ask the right questions, and to play at least one part, though perhaps not an official one, in helping the department's decision-making procedures on new applicants.

Some of our suggestions were not implemented for various reasons, not the least being practical considerations in terms of time, effort, and staff available on the part of the agency to engage in developing the foster parents group. The department was also limited by rules and regulations governing public agencies as well as by political realities which made it difficult, if not impossible, to implement the suggestion of using foster parents as screeners or advisors for new applicants. However, the agency did proceed in the development of a foster parents organization, held several general meetings and some small regional meetings. The foster parents themselves were eager to organize and developed their own initiative in terms of electing officers, held some meetings on their own, and positively responded to the notion of developing a closer relationship to the administration and the agency.

One of the advantages of being allowed to participate in some of the discussions and planning around this sort of program was that the consultants were then in a position to inquire about the progress of the program without such an inquiry being viewed as intrusive or meddling. Consultants should recognize in both program and administrative consultation, that they are consultants. They have neither the obligations nor the responsibilities of the actual administrators of the agency, who have to respond to expectations from various sources: staff, clients, superiors, and for a public agency, politicians. Consultants should avoid the grandiosity of "sit lux erat lux." (See glossary Table 1.1.) Consultants are sideliners; they are extraneous; they are expendable. If they construe their role as fomenters of abrupt change, as in recent times many so-called change agents have done, then they must be ready to pay the price of rapidly becoming former consultants whose mistakes someone else has to clean up.

A second example of a combination of administrative and program consultation concerned the issue of temporary care. Case consultation, which focused on certain recurrent experiences of particular children, served as a means of detecting general mental health risks to which large numbers of foster children are exposed. One such risk is that of temporary placement. The notion of temporary placement communicates to child, parent, and worker: "Don't invest; don't get too involved with each other." Prolonged temporary placement is a psychological bind. Multiple temporary placements increase the vulnerability of the child to development of an affectionless superficial style of relating. Such a child distrusts adults, expects disappointment, learns to use others instrumentally, often incorporates an image of himself as bad or unwanted, and frequently has recurrent depressive episodes.

From early in the consultation program, the consultants expressed their concern about this problem in the planning and review sessions. Our concern struck a responsive chord in the concerns of the administration of the department. For a long time, the director and her cabinet had been dissatisfied with the situation of temporary placement. Though hampered by lack of funds, personnel, and an inadequate supply of foster parents, the agency did initiate an alternative approach to this type of placement. It established several homes which were to provide definitive continuous placement for children immediately after their intake into care. The foster parents of these homes received intensive casework support from a worker exclusively assigned to this task. In this instance, the consultation effort was both administrative and programmatic. We helped the agency examine its procedures and policies; we identified the mental health issues involved in the present approach, and we supported their proposed modification as well as aiding in the planning of the new program. Several times we were asked to discuss certain problems in implementing the new approach, and we provided consultative help to the worker and her supervisor in their intensive work with these selected foster families.

MODEL FOR CONSULTATION

One of the goals of the original consultation agreement was to develop a model for mental health consultation in a public welfare agency. Though such a model is never definitive and should always be subject to revision and change, the opinion of the consultants and the agency was that the general outlines and components required of a useful model had been developed. (The two specific agency activities, II. A and B, designated below had not been implemented, however.) In the previous sections, we have essentially described the in vivo model building which derived from our ongoing experience. The components of the model are specifically applicable to our work in the welfare agency. However, we believe that its structured approach is general enough to be useful with modification in other large agencies and institutions such as schools, group living centers, delinquent settings, and child care programs.

MODEL

I. Consultant activities
    A. Case consultation
    B. Emergency service
    C. Direct evaluation and treatment services
    D. Advocacy, referral, and linking services (The consultant uses his knowledge

and contacts to expedite referral and appropriate services for a child when the casework staff encounters bureaucratic barriers to such referral.)

E. Planning and review function

F. Program and administrative consultation

G. Staff development

II. Agency activities (Various levels of the agency staff will, of course, be intimately involved with various consultant activities listed above. In addition, however, the agency has the opportunity to develop some specific mental health-related components of its own within this model.)

A. Mental health intervention group (This group could be composed of five to eight workers and a supervisor. They would receive some inservice training from the mental health consultants through the training component listed above. The function of this group would be to provide some screening and review of cases with the consultant. For some cases, a member of this group would provide intensive crisis intervention for a limited time. This could be provided by a worker under the direction of the supervisor or the consultants themselves. Weekly meetings of the intervention group could be held to review and discuss the status of various cases. The workers in this group would have a reduced regular caseload. When working on a crisis situation, they would not replace the regular caseworker but would offer supplementary help focused on the foster child, the parents, the natural family, or whatever other aspect of the case was identified as the point of intervention and support. Such an approach, or one like it, has the advantage of amplifying the effect of the mental health professional and of enhancing the skills of the caseworkers—an absolute necessity if they are to cope with the range of problems presented to a department of welfare. It would be useful to rotate some of the members of the crisis team or mental health intervention group so that new staff could be trained and developed while maintaining some stability in the structure of the team by continuing some members as permanent.)

B. Liaison or mediational personnel (This component would include liaison or mediational personnel to schools, courts, health centers, and other institutions which are intimately involved in the lives of children in placement. Some liaison personnel could also function as members of the mental health intervention team described above. However, since functions are quite different, one being crisis-oriented and the other a more ongoing administrative function, it would probably be best if the personnel of these two components were different. It would, however, be quite important for the supervisors in each of these two components to be in close contact and to be part of the administrative and review sessions in regular contact with the consulting professionals.)

REFERENCES

1. Eisenberg L, Marlowe B, Hastings M: Diagnostic services for maladjusted foster children: an orientation toward an acute need. Am J Orthopsychiatry 28:750–763, 1958
2. Wolkind S, Rutter M: Children who have been "in care"—an epidemiologic study. J Child Psychol Psychiatry 14:97–107, 1973
3. Young L: Wednesday's Children. New York, McGraw-Hill, 1964
4. Bowlby J: Attachment. New York, Basic Books, 1969
5. Hughes E: Good people and dirty work. Soc Probl 10:3–11, 1962
6. Rainwater L: Revolt of the dirty workers. Transaction 5:2, 64, 1967
7. Ormsby R: Group psychiatric consultation in a family casework agency. Soc Casework 31:361–365, 1950
8. Bernard V: Psychiatric Consultation in the social agency. Child Welfare 33:3–8, 1954
9. U.S. Dept. Health, Education, and Welfare, Social Security Administration, Children's Bureau: Rosenthal MJ, Sullivan ME: Psychiatric Consultation in a Child Public Welfare Agency. Washington D.C., U.S. Govt. Printing Office, 1959
10. Berne E: Games People Play: The Psychology of Human Relationships. New York, Grove, 1964, p 124
11. Berne E: Games People Play: The Psychology of Human Relations. New York, Grove, 1964, pp 110–112
12. Offer D: The Psychological World of the Teen-Ager: A Study of Normal Adolescent Boys. New York, Basic Books, 1969
13. White RW: Motivation reconsidered: the concept of competence. Psychol Rev 66:297–333, 1959
14. Caplan G: Theory and Practice of Mental Health Consultation. New York Basic Books, 1970
15. U.S. Dept. Health, Education, and Welfare Public Health Service, Health Services and Mental Health Administration: McClung FB, Stunden AA: Mental Health Consultation to Programs for Children. Washington, D.C., U.S. Govt. Printing Office, 1970

Part III

New Manpower Resources

8

Parent Education Program

We wish to educate and train primary caregivers who spend time with children to be more effective in their roles. The obvious and preeminent primary caregiver is the parent. Among the various actions and behaviors of being a parent, it is possible to distinguish or categorize several roles. There is the set of nurturant behaviors that involve the parent in providing food, clothing, shelter, warmth, affection, and support. There is a set of executive or management behaviors concerned with setting physical limits to protect the child from harm, setting social limits, rewarding acceptable and punishing unacceptable behaviors, and guiding the child through his daily round of activities. There are also those behaviors which are essentially tutorial and instructional in both the formal and informal sense. These include behaviors which essentially impart information about the world, interpret the child's experience, and help provide names and labels for persons, things, and events. These activities enable the child to make sense of the world and to gain useful knowledge from his experience which prepares him to use that experience in an anticipatory and predictive way. It then becomes obvious that parents are the first essential and most continuous teachers of their children, not only in the infancy and preschool period but throughout the school years into adolescence, and in some

We wish to acknowledge the work of Christine Kennedy, M.A., and Millie Thompson Bailey in the development and implementation of this program and for providing the curricular extracts cited.

ways, after emancipation. The teaching, of course, involves both prescription and proscription, both word and deed. There is much evidence in the developmental literature to support the effectiveness of modeling behavior by significant adults on the subsequent behavior of children.[1-4]

Our clinical impression and observation has been that mothers who live in poverty areas differentially emphasize one set of role behaviors over another. Thus, the nurturant and executive or management roles are generally more explicitly and intentionally developed than the teaching role. We believed that a program designed to help mothers become aware of their inherent teaching role would be useful in several ways. It would enhance the kind, quality, and goal directedness of certain interactions of the mother with her preschool child. It would promote the child's social and cognitive skill development and hopefully prepare him to become a more effective learner when he entered school. It would help improve the mutually interesting and interested child-parent relationship around some specific tasks and activities. The enhancement of the mother's competence in her teaching role would additionally improve her own self-esteem. She would then feel more effective in negotiating with the school system when her child was in school in the future. So often, all parents, but particularly parents from poor areas who have limited formal education and low-paying jobs, find themselves in a one-down position, both in their own minds and in the minds of teachers and school personnel. This low status position decreases their effective bargaining power and their confidence in asserting their concerns regarding the education of their children. Further, it tends to minimize the confidence they feel in transmitting their own knowledge and experience to their child. They often defer to the teacher as expert, not only in teaching matters but in other respects with their child. We wanted to encourage and promote in every possible way that parents were, in fact, the experts when it came to their own children.

Many of the compensatory or remedial education programs of the sixties have been child centered.[5] Although these programs have often had good rationales and results, they also displayed both conceptual and practical limitations. They tend to leave the parent out, put the parent on the sideline, and essentially the child is taken over by experts. Often parents are quite willing for this to happen, both for instrumental and expediency purposes, and also because of their own feelings of ineffectiveness and inadequacy in the teaching role. If one does not see onself as a teacher of one's own child, then one automatically does not feel confident or able to carry out tasks that are essentially teaching tasks. We were further concerned with the long-range effect that had been the experience of the second generation of immigrant populations to this country. Children of immigrant Germans, Poles, Italians, Greeks, Jews, and Irish had become acculturated to the American society primarily through the vehicle of the school system. Accompanying this acculturation came the rejection of the old parent culture and with it, frequently, the rejection of the parents themselves. We felt that to whatever degree a child-centered program focused on the children of the poor, it eliminated and excluded parents from the central interactions and concerns of the program. To this degree, one ran the risk of children subsequently becoming somewhat alienated from their parents. Since the whole fabric of family life among the poor is often tenuous, a program which might further rend this fabric, however good its intentions, would cost too high a price in human terms. From a very practical point of view, most of the child-centered programs only dealt with children for a few hours a day. When one considers the relative weight that these few hours have compared to the much longer period of time when the child is involved with his home environment, a very realistic case can be made for involving the parents as much as possible in the central aspects of any program.

The concept of high risk or vulnerability can be applied to preschool children from poor areas. Many of them are vulnerable and at high risk for subsequent school failure. There is an extensive literature on the cause and locus of this failure, whether genetic, parental, educational, socioeconomic, or otherwise.[6-9] The facts are that poor children by the fourth and fifth grade are doing less well academically than children from working and middle class families at the same grade level.[10] In addition, a relative scale of risk exists among the poor children.

We wanted to direct our program to those parents and children who were at a relatively high risk even within the poor population. We determined that one group of such children might be those who are eligible for, but would not get into preschool programs such as Get Set and Head Start. It was clear that parents who had the initiative and capacity for foresight and planning to enroll their children were different from parents who cannot or who do not succeed in this endeavor. The hardest to reach are those who may not even know about such a program or who may be so apathetic or overwhelmed by other priorities that they cannot generate the motivation to get involved. We struggled to think of ways to reach the hardest to reach; we did not come up with any effective methods. Therefore, we decided to try to involve those who were not formally enrolled in such preschool programs but who had shown enough interest to sign up and who were on waiting lists.

Any effective mental health program should be parsimonious in terms of its use of time and people, and should be capable of amplification and multiplication. Each of these features should be built into the design. We wanted, therefore, to design parent education groups so that they required the least possible expenditure of professional time, supplies, and expenses, without in any way impeding their educational goals. We thus wanted a program that was not merely another expensively operated pilot project in which large numbers of professionally trained and highly salaried people worked with a relatively small number of children. We wanted to develop a program that had components in terms of people, supplies, and expenses that could be adapted to reach all possible users in a population. Get Set Programs and Head Start Programs, as useful as they were, were still relatively expensive. Even at the time we conceived of this program (in the midsixties when in retrospect a comparatively large amount of federal money was being devoted to social welfare), it was still clear that the priorities throughout the war in Vietnam did not lie in human service programs. Given the present administration's surgical approach in terms of complete amputation for some programs and significant reduction in financial blood supply for others producing gradual atrophy and death, it is clear that any approach which is to have a chance at survival necessitates parsimony in the extreme.

INITIAL PILOT PROJECT

Through contact with the local Get Set Centers and the central Get Set Office, we determined that there was at least one child on a waiting list for every child in a Get Set Center. Many of these children will never get into Get Set because of the shortage of funds and staff. At the time we developed the program, there were 5,000 local children who were receiving the advantage of the formal Get Set Program. There were an additional 5,000 who were waiting on the doorstep and might never get in. In addition to those on the waiting list, there were uncounted thousands more children whose mothers had not been motivated to register and to wait, or who had not been reached and recruited by the program.

In the design of our program, we were influenced by several well-known workers in the area of preschool education, child development, and parent education.[11-17] We cannot review their contributions here, but their ideas form the substrate of our intervention efforts.

The initial pilot project was started in a Get Set Center in a Lutheran church building across the street from the Community Mental Health Center. Two members of the Children and Family Unit staff, a group specialist with experience in community organization, and a mental health assistant were our primary organizers. The director of the Children and Family Unit and a staff psychologist served as consultants and advisors.

We specifically chose a community building rather than using available space in the mental health center. First, we wished to use the structure that members of the community used for some of their own activities. Second, since this was a promotional or positive mental health program, we wanted to avoid any possible stigma that might be attached to parents and children if they came to a mental health center which in their minds had been established to treat emotionally ill children. Since our population of children was selected from the normal population, we felt that working in an established community center would be the most logical and natural strategy. In addition, we wanted to demonstrate our concern about positive mental health intervention and to attempt to broaden the conception in the community's mind of what mental health was all about. We thus wanted to avoid as much as possible the exclusive association with the concept of hospital, clinic, or place where illness and disease are treated.*

The staff of the mental health center contacted the parents of children who were on the waiting list for this particular Get Set Center. We did this through letters, phone calls, and face-to-face visiting. With the help of the staff of the Get Set Center, the Children and Family Unit staff arranged for an introductory and explanatory meeting to present the aims, goals, and procedures of the program to interested mothers and fathers. Twenty mothers attended the introductory meeting. Members of the staff of the Get Set program served as cohostesses with two or three waiting-list mothers who had been particularly eager and interested to become involved. Initially, coffee and rolls were served and people began to socialize with each other. Following this introduction, the Children and Family Unit staff members explained the purpose of the meeting and the plans for parent education sessions. Next came a discussion period in which parents asked questions, offered suggestions, and the staff of the mental health center responded. Ten parents indicated their willingness to participate and future meetings were established for Monday afternoons. Arrangements were made so that parents could bring their preschool children with them, not only the index child but any younger children. The staff of the

*This is a significant and central issue in overall mental health strategy and planning. It touches on such matters as whether mental health centers should be free standing or part of multiservice centers or comprehensive health operations. It also brings into question the medical health-illness model versus the social developmental or adaptational model, and the theoretical as well as practical implications of these models. Further, it tends to contrast the initiating versus the responding type of approach, or the structural versus the functional approach to mental health programs. The latter distinction is to highlight that most mental health services are given inside a mental health structure, clinic, or hospital where patients come to be treated and helped. The functional approach is manifested by programs in which the mental health staff reaches out to a population and moves into institutions that serve the population. This means that the actual staff of the mental health center works in a neighborhood or community institution such as school, recreation center, settlement house, or health center. Mental health programs need both types of approach, but there has been too much emphasis in the past on the structural responding mode as opposed to the functional initiating mode.

mental health center had recruited students from Temple University Child
Care Training Program to spend time engaging the children in useful and
enjoyable activities while their mothers would meet with the mental health
center staff in the parent education sessions.

The program as presented to the parents at the first meeting included
the following goals:

1. To establish and promote increased opportunities for communication
   and understanding among parents and between parents and their
   children;
2. To increase participation by parents in their children's education, both
   as educators in the early and preschool years and then later as
   interested advocates, consumers, and negotiators with school personnel;
3. To increase the parents' knowledge and experience in childrearing
   methods and in certain particular techniques of enhancing the
   children's learning;
4. To bring practical help to parents in preparing play material and planning activities for children;
5. By several of the above goals, hopefully to promote effective school
   performance by the children when they enter school;
6. To increase self-esteem of parents, particularly by enhancing their
   awareness of their role as primary teachers and educators of their own
   children, as well as by increasing their repertoire of teaching skills and
   activities.

The initial pilot group met weekly for a period of 10 weeks. After an
orientation discussion, the parents were shown a slide show of various
preschool situations. Subsequent workshops were held on reading
readiness, math readiness, puzzle solving, educational games, and
children's art. Verbal skills were particularly stressed in the interchange
between mother and child. Materials were used which were either
naturally occurring in most homes or could be obtained at little or no cost.
These included shoeboxes, plastic food containers, paper bags, news-
papers, egg cartons, and other common household items. The content of
the workshops had been developed from a fairly extensive review of the
literature and after consultation with local experts in the field.

Field trips were undertaken by the children and parents to local mu-
seums, supermarkets, and schools. Neighborhood walks, in which a premium was put on observing, naming, and discussing common events,
persons, or places encountered on the way, were used to promote parent-
child verbal interaction as well as to increase the child's observational

skills and to orient him to the particular characteristics of his neighborhood. Discussions about childrearing problems with the child psychiatric consultant were carried out. During the time that the parents and group leaders spent together, the university students not only provided recreation to the children but reinforced with them some of the learning skills and tasks that were used in the workshops.

The first workshop pilot program led to the development of a curriculum which is outlined below and is described as Parent Workshop Series I.

I. Session I
    A. Slide presentation: preschoolers learn at play
    B. High chair games
        1. Counting box—math concepts: categorizing, counting, arranging in size order
        2. Stringing beads, spools, macaroni-counting, learning colors, practicing manipulative skills
        3. Group ideas and discussion
II. Session II
    A. Demonstration of Session I materials with children: group members participate.
    B. Verbal development of children
        1. Games while dressing, feeding, bathing; learn common greetings, parts of body, names of things
        2. Tones of the language; have "conversations"; do not talk "at" children too much; talk then becomes only a noise, not a meaningful, directed communication.
        3. Have experiences; converse about them.
        4. Songs, rhythm games
        5. Group ideas and discussion
III. Session III
    A. Finger painting: the development of children's art.
    B. Group discussion and participation; wear washable clothing or smocks.
IV. Session IV
    A. Behavior: what is a "good" child? We will share our viewpoints. There are no "experts" who know the answers for *your* child as well as you.
    B. We will each make a sock puppet. Bring a worn out sock if you have one. Do not bring a new one. Puppets are fun and also help a child talk about things in make believe that are too scary or doubtful to talk about for real.
V. Session V
    A. Feel box: a guessing game teaching sense of touch and descriptive skills
    B. Demonstration by members of verbal games with their children

VI.   Session VI
A.   Puzzles: teach geometric shapes, pictures of things, manipulative control, reasoning skills
B.   Things older brothers and sisters can make for baby
1.   Make mobiles for cribs.
2.   Paint and label shoeboxes for storage.
3.   Make large word cards to put on common house items, such as sink, bed, and other items.
C.   Discussion and evaluation of the workshops. How can the group continue to share their ideas and become better teachers of their children?

As we planned the program, the members of the staff of the mental health center agreed that the leaders would not involve themselves in teaching the children directly. After an initial demonstration of the particular content of the session, carried out by the leaders with the parents alone, the parents and children then met all together. For the next hour or so, the parent worked with one of her children individually. The staff were involved only as observers and guides, helping the mothers in teaching their children. This teaching was done circumspectly and carefully so as to preserve the resourcefulness and unique approach that each parent had with her own child and to diminish the parent's anxiety or uncertainty as she demonstrated a new activity. It was apparent from the start that helping the mothers become comfortable with each other and developing a group spirit and identity in which they shared their successes and also their failures without shame, facilitated each mother's work with her own child when they met as a total group. The leaders found that those mothers who had anxiety about their performance because of the fear of embarrassment in front of the other mothers could be helped not only by the leaders but particularly by the other mothers' encouragement, suggestions, and recognition.

Both the relationships developed in the group and the common task orientation promoted a more general sense of sociability and comfort which extended to activities outside the formal sessions. This was, in part, related to the fact that the mothers lived close to each other. In addition, their children would be attending the same kindergarten the following year. They thus found not only common interests in the present but the possibility of common interests in the future and in their children's educational experience. In fact, the original pilot group decided to continue their regular meetings throughout the summer without depending on the presence of a staff member.

In conjunction with a local parent-child center, we developed a similar program for mothers of children under the age of 3. The group leaders took notes of their sessions with the mothers, and the following are several extracts:

We began the math workshop by giving examples of the natural things around the house that we do that are related to math concepts: setting the table, passing out cookies, buttoning, and counting steps. We told the parents that by being aware of the value of talking about these routine and daily activities, and by encouraging the children to help them whenever they can, they not only get their work done but they teach as well.

We had one of the mothers get her 1.5-year-old child from the playroom and demonstrate with her the concept of big and little, as well as the differences or categories of things. We used some stones and small sticks and twigs. One of the characteristics of the interaction was the quality of warmth and mutual interest the child and mother displayed to each other. The mother held the little girl in her lap and praised her when she would "give mommy the big stick" or "the little one" or one of the stones. The mother had not planned the demonstration in advance and within three or four repetitions, the child had grasped all the directions given in the brief lesson.

In addition to the particular activities, the sessions focused on other serious and relevant concerns of the parents which were brought to the staff members.

While we were all working and painting together around the table, several mothers talked about their children. They seemed eager to ask questions of us about their older children's development, especially around school behavior and performance. One mother said a housing manager had remarked that her son seemed retarded and had suggested a special school. The mother seemed to be seeking someone to reassure her, but she said that she had never followed up on the person's suggestion. It was apparent that this had been on her mind a long time. The boy is now age 14 and it was 2 years ago that the remark by the housing manager was made. The group picked up on this in a responsive way. It was pointed out that the housing manager, although trying to be helpful, was not an expert on mental retardation. We said that many times children get labeled and that label affects their ability to achieve at their best. We also mentioned that if she still continued to be concerned about her son's possible retardation, there were clinics she could take him to for evaluation.

The staff provided some direct help with this and other situations. On occasion, they would see the child if necessary or discuss the problems with the concerned teacher or school staff. If they felt the need for further help, they would discuss the matter with a psychiatrist or psychologist from the Children and Family Unit. Direct referral for evaluation or follow-up care or planning for educational or other services could be carried out within the framework of the mental health center. Though, as stated above, the primary effort or intent of the program was not casefinding or identification, when the need arose, the staff was able to fill this function of getting mothers and children to needed services, and of providing advocacy, follow-up, and linkage where needed. Parents were helped to make connections to medical, welfare, and other services.

Concerns about child management and behavior were discussed at the sessions:

> The 2-year-old son of one of the group members was crying loudly upstairs for quite a long time. This prompted a brief discussion of ways to deal with a child's fears of separation from his mother. We stressed the importance of always telling the truth to your child, and never saying, "mommy's going to be there" when she is really going to sneak away. We suggested a verbal pattern of something that you say when you leave a child briefly, such as "I'll be back" and then for mother to reappear in a minute or so. This would set a pattern of secure expectation in the child so that when you leave him for longer periods he will feel safe.

The concrete activities that were demonstrated at each session often provided a springboard for a discussion of larger issues which had a direct bearing on emotional development and mental health:

> The task in the workshop this time was to paint and fill a "feel box." This is a shoebox with a hole cut in the top and with various items within the box that the child can feel and learn to describe. The items included cotton, sandpaper, a nail, a large marble, and a satin ribbon. The staff explained that this game can be used to develop connection between verbal skills and sensation of touch.

> The point of describing how things feel was carried into the realm of emotional feelings, and mothers were encouraged to say back to the child how he thinks he may be feeling. For example, we pointed out that if the child is making a frown and seems ready to cry or hit someone, mother can say "I bet you feel angry" or "I bet you feel like hitting your brother." Learning how to verbalize can help the child with his feelings as well as helping the mother understand him.

> In this session, two new members each demonstrated their boxes with their children after they had made them, and it was interesting to note how the veteran members instructed the new ones. For example, someone said, "Let him do it." when the mother was tempted to overdirect the child in his performance. Another member of the group said to a mother regarding the latter's child, "He's tired and doesn't want to do it in front of all of us."

> The mothers, when asked whether they were using the workshop materials replied in various ways. The concepts learned seemed to be used more than the actual workshop boxes. This may indicate that the major felt need of the group is to get together to discuss shared problems, feelings, and to have a degree of sociability. It also indicates that a way of following-up on helping persons is probably needed in the program design.

PLANS FOR AMPLIFICATION AND REPLICATION

Important criteria for mental health programs to meet include amplification, that is, where a small input results in a relatively larger output, and replication. As we conceived of the parent education program, it had the potential for fulfilling both. Having had the experience of carrying out three different programs, two with children over 3 and one with children under 3, each representing a modification and an improvement over the previous one, the staff was prepared to proceed to develop a more elaborate and extensive program in conjunction with the School District of Philadelphia. We planned to recruit several of the mothers that had participated in the previous workshops, and to provide them with leadership training experience so that they could conduct parent education groups similar to the ones that our staff had conducted with them. We saw the leadership training as a three-step arrangement. First, there would be individual tutorial and supervisory meetings between our staff and the parents who had been selected from the previous groups. Second, the leaders in training would be assigned to work with our staff in several parent education workshops, first as observers, but soon as participant coleaders. This work would be supplemented by discussions of group dynamics and group formation; that is, how to establish goals for a group, and how to keep a group task-oriented while still encouraging informality in the discussion of feelings and ideas. Further, the potential leaders would learn how to present the teaching materials and to demonstrate to parents how they could use them with their own children. The overall object would be exactly the same; that is, the parent group leaders would not be the primary teachers of the children, but the members of the group would be shown how and what to do. They, in turn, would practice throughout the week with the materials, and return the next week for new workshop materials.

Because the leaders in training would be recruited from the parents who had been involved in the earlier projects, the local neighborhood community character of the program would be maintained. We would encourage the parent leaders who were trained to recruit new parents who lived in or near the community, whether or not they used the particular facility. Thus, over a period of several workshops, a sizable number of parents and families could be reached in a local area. At this point in time, the staff of the mental health center would be serving more as consultants, advisors, and trouble shooters. In conjunction with the newly trained parent leaders, they would review each workshop series in order to improve the curriculum, incorporating suggestions from the parent leaders or parent participants.

As an alternative approach, we also presented the School District of Philadelphia with a plan in which home and school coordinators and parents would work together as coleaders to carry out a parent education workshop series in a number of local schools.* The home and school coordinator in each school would recruit one parent of a 4-year-old scheduled to attend that school in the future. This parent would enter our training program, and would subsequently become a parent group leader and School District employee if, during her training, she proved she had the ability and skills to be successful in this job. Through such a plan, the school would have participated in the development of informed, articulate, confident, and competent parent educators, who by reason of their concern and skills could be useful in promoting educational improvement for all children in the school, as well as for their own. They could serve as a nucleus to generate and encourage other parents' interests not only at the preschool level but throughout the elementary school years.

It is relevant to note at this point that when interviewing a number of young adults for the position of incentive specialists (see Chapter 11), one question invariably brought the same general answer from every applicant. When asked why they had successfully persisted until they had completed high school, while so many of their classmates had dropped out, these young adults invariably mentioned the personal influence of a parent, aunt, grandparent, or teacher close to them throughout childhood who believed in them and who stressed the importance of educational achievement. Although such a statement can be dismissed as Blinding Glimpse into the Obvious #8147, it is often overlooked and obscured by the increasing stockpiling of curricular revisions, programmed methods, team teaching,

---

*The home and school coordinator is a role created for urban schools in poverty areas. The coordinator, a paid school employee, was intended to be a parent or other community resident who would function to enhance mutual understanding and communication between the school and the local community which it served. The actual tasks that the coordinator carried out varied widely according to the way in which a particular principal envisioned the role. Some home and school coordinators were very actively involved in work in the community and informed the school of parents' interests and complaints and generated meetings in homes between parents and school staff. They also followed-up on referrals from counselors and teachers on children who might be having problems in school attendance. Other coordinators were merely sideline operators who were used in a narrow and restricted way, kept within the school building and not allowed to promote closer coordination between school staff and parents. There is a tendency for such jobs in poor areas to be treated as patronage positions, to be jealously sought after, and to be used as sources of personal or group power against a competing person or community group. The scarcity of these and similar positions in both the public and private sector in poor communities frequently elicited from the possessor of the job a degree of defensiveness, guardianship of prerogatives, and status consciousness that were frequently derided as being the sole possession of bureaucrats and professionals.

open classrooms, and other such innovations. What is propounded in doctoral theses, hopefully with a fair amount of scientific reserve and objectivity, is frequently rushed into mass production by the educational developmental labs and curriculum factories that have sprung up with a rapidity and density matched only by drive-in eateries. This can lead to some of the more blatant, simplistic forms of the new hucksterism that appeared in the educational fields in the fifties and sixties.

· At times, it is important to return to the basics, to reassert them, and to develop programs that will promote and encourage such obviously important processes. For these young people who are interested in becoming incentive specialists, an interested, concerned, responsive, and available adult had been the significant factor in their educational success and in their life success up to that point. This was exactly the kind of natural process that we hoped to build on and to develop in our parent education program. We were convinced the school had an investment in the same process, given the repeated assertion that parental involvement is crucial if schools are to be successful in their task with children.

FAILURE AND SURVIVAL STRATEGIES

What happened to our proposal? Very simply, it died aborning. The immediate cause of death was acute insufficiency of the green folding stuff which nurtures and sustains the just and unjust alike. Its more remote cause was the same virus responsible for the death of so many programs: "It's a good idea, but. . . ."

Of the lack of funds, we can make a generalization. Whenever an administrator says, "That's a good idea, but we don't have funds to support it at this time," you can be sure that either you as the huckster of the program or the program itself has a relatively low priority in the administrator's scale of things he wants to do or get done. This low priority may be attributed to a number of factors, excluding personality clashes or problems between the administrator and the program presenter. Two major dimensions or issues around which many of the reservations of an administrator may cluster are those of usefullness and feasibility. If his reservations center on the first issue, usefullness, the task of the program promoter in changing the administrator's mind is the more difficult one. If, however, it is essentially feasibility (and often feasibility is a camouflage for the administrator's true view that the program is useless and not valuable to him), the mental health salesman's job is somewhat easier and has to do with his skill in persuading the administrator to consider various practical approaches to implementing the program.

As to altering an administrator's decision when his own set of beliefs are quite at variance with the program's goals such that he does not see its intrinsic or potential usefullness, there are a more limited number of alternatives. One obvious approach is to find some congruence between the administrator's set of values and those of the program one is promoting. For example, in the parent education program, one school administrator was not particularly interested in preschool education, nor was he particularly impressed with the notion that parents are able to be teachers of their children. Having been a teacher himself and valuing the professional role of the teacher, he thought the program represented a devaluation of this role. He essentially saw teaching by parents as meddling in an area in which they were not competent. Perhaps, they would confuse the child and make him less prepared for school, and because of possible confusion, the parent may create more resistance to learning. However, this same administrator was very interested in promoting closer cooperation between the community and school. He wished to develop an active home and school association and was enthusiastic about the potential usefullness of the home and school coordinator. The program we presented, in which the home and school coordinator and the parent would work together, attracted him because of its possible value in promoting closer school and community relationships with parents even before their children were in school. He thus became a supporter of the program because the program represented in some of its goals one of his high priorities. For us, this was an important, but secondary priority.

A second strategy for attempting to deal with a conflict in values between an administrator and a promoter is to find some way to honestly appeal to the administrator's enlightened self-interest. For example, agreeing to such a program would bring him increased personal prestige or increase his political leverage relative to other administrators, his superiors, community groups, or within the mental health field itself. Sometimes a new program might help put out some fires or help him with problems he may be having in some other aspect of his own program which is not going well. However, the promoter's attempt to use such leverage puts the program, once implemented, in a potentially dangerous position. If it turns out poorly, and leads to more difficulty for the administrator, then the program, its promoter, and its clients are all in trouble.

When there is a discrepancy between the promoter and the administrator about the value of a program, one strategy too frequently used by promoters is that of moral righteousness in an attempt to induce guilt. For instance, if an administrator did not particularly see the value in our parent education program, this strategy would call for the promoter to somehow imply that the administrator was against parenthood, was ignorant of the potential educability of the preschool child, was perhaps afraid of empowered and competent parents who could deal with the school effectively, and was even a classist or racist. Such techniques have often been used both in private negotiations and in public issues, and they are easily elaborated by the press and broadcast media. From a psychosocial view, most clinicians in the mental health field are aware that any triumph gained by asserting real or supposed moral superiority is in the long run, a Pyrrhic victory.

The parent education program suffered failure because of difficulties encountered both within the mental health center and in attempting to promote the program within the public school system. Additionally, mental health funding authorities were not at that time investing in programs of a preventive nature, whether preschool, consultative, or other such positive mental health interventions. These authorities tended to be interested in body count programs in which individual human beings, identified as patients, in some way pass a turnstile into a structure that is labeled mental health center, hospital, or clinic. They then can be counted and accounted for. This is essentially an administrative and fiscal approach to mental health services though it has largely been supported by medical and psychiatric tradition in terms of the provision of both inpatient and outpatient services.

Within the mental health center, a lack of interest and response resulted, in part, because the promoters of the program within the Children and Family Unit, including the director, did not attend carefully to the strategies appropriate to the issue of mismatched or competing priorities. The parent education program itself was not one that automatically touched central interests of the center. As it did not fall within the primary set of priorities, one again received the response, "it's a good idea, but. . . ." Had we been more sagacious, we could have included in our proposal some adult outpatients as participants in the parent education program. There were a number of adult patients who had preschool children and who could have been included along with parents recruited from the community. We also could have combined our efforts with a community involvement of the center's consultation and education unit. This group was attempting to work with local community development groups around a variety of mental health-related issues. Including our program as part of the consultation unit's work with a local community center could have been a way of encouraging a community group to sponsor a parent education group for adults who were members of their organization. Finally, in most mental health centers as they were in the sixties, and as they are today, most of the services are treatment-oriented. The parent education program is a positive mental health intervention program, which promotes adaptation and is directed toward nonsick persons who do not have any obvious clinical problems. From the viewpoint of those services that are primarily treatment or sickness-oriented, such a program as parent education can be seen as a luxury. In this light, mental health centers are, and have been, primarily mental illness treatment centers—attempting to restore persons to a mentally healthy state. In most instances, only lip service is paid to the positive programs aimed at promoting more effective mental health adaptation among at-risk, but not sick, groups.

We also failed in our efforts to gain the financial backing of the School District of Philadelphia in funding the proposal which would have used home and school coordinators and parents in developing parent education workshops. Several reasons were operative. The first was a matter of timing. The school district was at that time in the process of centralizing several of its programs which were directed toward preschool children. Some increased federal money was available and there was a reorganization to put all of these programs under one administrative director. In these circumstances, we learned a lesson that is perhaps generally useful. When a system or institution is reorganizing and undergoing a fair amount of change with confusion and dislocation of persons and programs, it is a bad time to try to interest it in sponsoring an outside program. Persons newly appointed to positions of power are reluctant to commit themselves to outside endeavors when they do not have their own house in order, or they are not yet secure in their new position. Old administrators who may be remaining are uncertain as to what the new alignments of power will be, and are unlikely to make new commitments. Old and new "yes" and "no" sayers will be hesitant to make decisions at a time of reorganization because most of their energies are directed internally. In addition, the eyes of their directors are on them, and they are concerned with protecting themselves and establishing the right impression. Thus, any new program which might turn out to be a failure, especially when it is being promoted and run by people outside the main system, will hardly be given a fair hearing at such a time.

Finally, the school, like other long-standing institutions, is heavy with tradition. A child-centered approach is the tradition of schools. Schools are not used to thinking of parents as partners in the teaching situation. Most school personnel do not really accept the notion of the parent as teacher. Their view of the parent is much like that of the professional viewing the amateur, or the physician viewing the patient who attempts to treat himself. Because the professional has invested so much time and effort in his own education, he feels that skills and knowledge which he has acquired are his exclusive right. Anyone else who tries to exercise them, and has not gone through the same experience or ritual, is at best muddle-headed and at worst pernicious. Schools during the sixties (and even today) were not ready to work closely with parents under "new contracts." The old contract applied in which parents could be helpful and cooperative, could join home and school associations, could come to meetings when asked, and could listen to the teachers talk. They were not to influence school policy or curriculum, or in any way intrude on the professional prerogatives of the school, teachers, and administrators.

In addition to this traditional view about parents, there was a markedly heightened anxiety on the part of school personnel in the mid and late sixties. The source of this anxiety was the increased activism of community groups regarding the issue of community control of schools. There had been several dramatic confrontations, particularly one in New York at Brownsville, and the problem had been simmering in Philadelphia. School administrators and teachers feared that parents would be too active and militant. The power of the teachers union had increased, and the teachers saw the union as a refuge, both from the administrators, as well as from the growing threat of community control groups. Into this mix, the perennial issues of race and class entered. In urban areas, poor black and Puerto Rican children were the predominant consumers of public school education. Because the school had failed to successfully educate these children, many of them were falling farther and farther behind national averages in achievement tests and thousands on thousands were dropping out of school in junior high school and beyond. The parents were anxious, disappointed, and angry. They saw their children being educationally disenfranchised and by this disenfranchisement being relegated to second-and third-class citizenship for the rest of their lives. This issue was only one of a number of larger issues of racial and class frustration around housing, unemployment, and police abuse that led to riots in many center city areas.

In such a climate, it is understandable that school personnel, particularly administrators, would be very wary about committing themselves to any program in which they would actively promote the organization of parent groups, even those devoted to such a laudable aim as education of preschool children. When the level of anxiety is high, there is a tendency for those who are apprehensive to generalize from the rare event. Teachers would cite an instance in which a parent came into the school, threatened the teacher, and caused a variety of disturbances. This became the image they then would see whenever they thought of parent involvement. If one would take the trouble to ask the teacher or principals who cited such an example how often in the past 5 years such an event had happened, one would find that it may have occurred once or twice in a given school in that period of time. But this is a typical example of living according to the law that the worst will still be the most probable. Our program, though quite an innocuous one in intent and method, raised the specter of parents organizing, becoming more vocal, more knowledgeable, and attempting to "try to tell the school how to do their job." All of these factors and others of which we are probably not aware led to the early neonatal death of the parent education program. It is encouraging to note that in the seventies, early childhood programs received new emphasis, essentially as a result of the widespread interest in development of day care centers.

REFERENCES

1. Bandura A, Walters RH: Social Learning and Personality Development. New York, Holt 1963
2. Hess RD, Shipman VC: Early experience and the socialization of cognitive modes in children. Child Dev 36:869–886, 1965
3. Kagan J, Moss H: Birth to Maturity. New York, Wiley, 1962
4. Sears RR, Maccoby EE, Levin H: Patterns of Child Rearing. Evanston, Row, Peterson, 1957
5. Caldwell BM: Impact of interest in early cognitive stimulation. In Rie HE (ed): Perspectives in Child Psychopathology. Chicago, Aldine-Atherton, Inc, 1971, pp 293–334
6. Bronfenbrenner U: The psychological costs of quality and equality in education. Child Dev 38:909–925, 1967
7. Coleman JS et al: Equality of Educational Opportunity. U.S. Dept. Health, Education, and Welfare, Office of Education. Washington, D.C., U.S. Govt. Printing Office, 1966
8. Deutsch M, Katz I, Jensen A: Social Class, Race and Psychological Development. Holt, 1968
9. Gray SW, Klaus RA: An experimental preschool program for culturally deprived children. Child Dev 36:887–898, 1965
10. Deutsch M: Minority groups and class status as related to social and personality factors in scholastic achievement. In Deutsch M (ed): Disadvantaged Child. New York, Basic Books, 1967, pp 89–132
11. Biber B, Franklin MB: The relevance of developmental and psychodynamic concepts to the education of the preschool child. In Hellmuth J (ed): The Disadvantaged Child, vol. I. Seattle, Special Child Publications, 1967, pp 305–323
12. Caldwell B, Richmond, J: The children's center in Syracuse, New York. In Dittman LL Early Child Care: The New Perspectives. New York, Atherton, 1968, pp 326–358
13. Gordon I: Early Child Stimulation through Parent Education: A Final Report to the Children's Bureau. Gainesville, Univ. Florida Press, 1969

14. Levenstein P, Sunley R: Stimulation of verbal interaction between disadvantaged mothers and children. Am J Orthopsychiatry 38:116–121, 1968
15. Levin T: Preschool education and the communities of the poor. In Hellmuth J (ed): Disadvantaged Child, vol. I. Seattle, Special Child Publications, 1967, pp 349–406
16. Schaefer ES: A home tutoring program. Children 16:59–61, 1969
17. Weikart D, Lambie D: Preschool intervention through a home teaching program. In Hellmuth J (ed): Disadvantaged Child, vol II. New York, Brunner/Mazel, 1968, pp 435–500

Glenn Taylor
Robert J. Stewart
Marc A. Forman

9

The Black Brother Program

Two black boys are sitting on a step in front of a house in North Philadelphia. The neighborhood meets the standard sociological criteria of a "ghetto"; abandoned homes, joblessness, high crime rate, many families on public assistance. The older boy, age 15, describes how he has just made the high school football team, after he had felt his chances were slim. At first, he had thought he might be a defensive end, but when his coach said he was too light, he agreed to be a corner linebacker. The younger boy, age 8, listens. He thinks it's neat; he'd settle for corner linebacker any day. He asks the older boy about how long he practices, what it involves, and who else is on the team. The older boy explains and says he'll show him some of the moves he recently learned.

Contrast this scene with that of another 8-year-old sitting in a psychiatrist's office in a local child guidance center. The boy is not sure why he is there, except that it may have something to do with trouble at school. The psychiatrist, white and about the same age as his school principal, is asking him whether he remembers his father who left home 4 years ago. The boy replies that he can't remember anything and wonders if that's the right answer to give. Perhaps, if he keeps saying that, the psychiatrist won't ask him any more questions.

These two examples are not given with the aim of romanticizing the first and denegrating the second. They serve as an introduction to the

We gratefully acknowledge the United Fund of Philadelphia for its financial support of the Black Brother Program.

Black Brother Program—a program based on the assumption that what occurred in the first situation could be just as "therapeutic," or even more so, than what happened in the second. The program attempts to use informal modeling experiences which occur between younger and older boys to help children who come from fatherless and broken homes.

What are the statistics and psychological sequelae of father-absence? The U.S. Office of Child Development[1] reported in 1971 that 8 million children were in fatherless homes. Possibly three times that number will experience this status, for shorter or longer periods, some time between birth and age 18. Information obtained from the Philadelphia 1970 Census, analyzed by the Philadelphia City Planning Commission, indicates that approximately 20 percent of the family household units in the city have a female head, while an additional 5 to 6 percent of the homes are headed by nonhusband males.

Literature representing the research on the effects of father-absence on boys is limited. Trends can be discerned, though the overall pattern is complex, and occasionally, contradictory.

Many of the effects often presumed to result from paternal-absence can largely be attributed to certain parental characteristics (intense conflict, rejection, and deviance) which occur more commonly in broken families.[2] Biller[3] suggests that the effects of father-absence on the personality development of the male child cannot be considered in isolation from other factors such as the length and timing of father-absence, the sociocultural milieu, the availability of surrogate models, and individual differences in maternal behavior.

Two of the more frequently used scales in studying father-absence are measures of masculinity-femininity and aggression. Santrock,[4] in a study of preschool father-absent children, found that father-absent (FA) children were significantly more feminine, less aggressive, and more dependent than father-present (FP) boys. In addition, FA boys whose older siblings were males only were significantly more masculine than FA boys with older female siblings only. On the dependency scale, FA boys with a father substitute were significantly less dependent than FA boys with no father substitute. Several related studies concluded that FA children who had one or more older male siblings were significantly more aggressive, less intensely dependent, and less frequently dependent than children who do not have older male siblings.[5,6] The presence of an older male sibling in the FA family appears to assist in making the FA child more like the child from the FP family. Other studies reveal that boys enduring a sustained period of father-absence are more likely to be socially immature, to be subject to greater peer rejection, and to be more emotionally maladjusted than father-present boys.[7,8]

As so often occurs in the scientific literature, there are also advocates of a somewhat different view. Herzog and Sudia[9] describe the methodological weaknesses in some studies on father-absence, point to the need to consider the child's total life situation, and cogently note that boys can still have contacts with adult males when there is not an intact marriage. A companion article by Herzog and Lewis[10] notes that "even if eventually a significant association can be demonstrated between father-absence and one of the adverse effects attributed to it, that impact is dwarfed by other factors in the interacting complex. Among these are the coping ability and individual makeup of the mother, especially her ability to give adequate mothering and supervision, the economic situation of the family, and community influences."

Even considering the lack of clarity in the studies, we feel it is reasonably safe to assert that father-absent boys are at-risk for the development of problems, especially those who come from homes in conflict and turmoil. In the ordinary course of events, many of these father-absent boys are referred to child psychiatric agencies. Their evaluations often include the phrase "needs masculine identification" and, as a corollary, "should have a male therapist." We agree that masculine identification is necessary for psychological growth, but there are ways of fostering it beyond psyychotherapeutic sessions with an adult male professional for 1 hour a week.

We know that young boys may be more influenced by teenagers than they are by adults. In various settings adolescents have been used as tutors and nursery school aides, and college-aged students have been employed as counselors. The gang system, ranging from the "old heads" down to the "mighty mites" and "peanuts" is a hierarchy built on the emulation of older youths by younger ones. Adolescents can be "cool dudes" while adults remain part of the "establishment" who want children to go to school, to learn and be obedient. But there are also adolescents who succeed within the prevailing value system, who go to school, who do not get into trouble, who maintain stable family relationships, and who have career goals. Why not use them as "therapists" and models for younger boys?

This conceptual shift led us to the development of the Black Brother Program. Our original program included the following goals:

1. To provide a different and more effective service model for black, latency age, father-absent boys who were experiencing emotional difficulties;
2. To provide male identification models for black, father-absent boys;
3. To help remediate behavioral and academic problems in father-absent boys;

4.. To train community personnel to become service providers;
5. More specifically, to create prevocational employment for community adolescents, and to introduce the area of mental health service as a possible future vocational choice.

To begin the program, the clinic director selected a young black male college graduate (G.T.) as the project director. He was in reality a paraprofessional, newly arrived at our agency and without any previous experience in a mental health facility. In many ways, he was grappling with clinical problems similar to those which our high school therapists would encounter. He essentially served as the teacher and model for our adolescent therapists (Big Brothers). Although he began as a novice, the project director felt his "newness" was an asset which he could share with the high school students in their new roles as "Big Brothers."

Next, two Big Brothers were selected from a class of a local all-male high school within walking distance from our clinic. We contacted the high school principal, explained our aims, and requested that he inform the students, counselors, and teachers about the program. The principal was also asked to screen a number of interested black students for subsequent interviews with the program director and clinic director. In choosing the Big Brothers we were looking for high school juniors, with a history of reasonably stable and reliable performance, who were in good academic standing, and who impressed us with their relational skills. Juniors were chosen because we felt that sophomores who were in their first year of high school might possibly be having adjustment problems and conflicts of their own. Seniors were apt to be very much involved in senior class activities, both academic and social, and might have been too occupied to give the required amount of time.

Initially, our rather intuitive selection process backfired and we had to drop our first two Big Brothers from the program after they failed to attend a number of the early orientation training sessions. We do not really know why there was this initial lack of an adequate fit between us and the first two Big Brothers. We do know that with our next two candidates, we were much more explicit, set firm limits, told them that they were embarking on a job which had definite and distinct responsibilities attached to it and explained that they would be dismissed if they could not meet those responsibilities. These two Big Brothers proved to be quite successful in their work.

In selecting the Little Brothers, we chose black, father-absent boys between the ages of 6 and 10 from our clinic's treatment waiting list. These boys had usually been referred by their school or families for behavioral or learning problems. They came from homes where there was no father, no older male sibling, and no other stable male available for identification and role modeling. Severely ego-impaired children or psychotic children were excluded. Each potential Little Brother was seen and his condition diagnosed through the regular clinic procedure. If it appeared that a child was not seriously disturbed but that he was having considerable adjustment difficulties and could benefit from a relationship with an older boy, the patient was referred to the Black Brother Program, and he then became the Little Brother.

We asked the Big Brothers to spend 10 hours per week with the Little Brothers doing almost any kind of activity that the pair mutually agreed on. They might go for walks, play football, do homework together, build models, or just talk. We paid the Big Brothers $2.00 per hour up to a maximum of $20.00 per week although some of the Big Brothers spent additional time with the Little Brother without further remuneration. The Big Brothers functioned as primary therapists. They were not cotherapists, auxiliary therapists, or junior therapists. This was the only form of therapy for the Little Brother, and their families had only intermittent contact with other clinic personnel. All the therapy between Big and Little Brothers was conducted outside of the clinic, in each other's homes, in the neighborhood, on the street.

Here is a live example of how John Jones, age 16, handled a problem with his Little Brother, Billy, age 8.

Billy didn't want to do his homework. He would just pick up his assignment book and leaf through it. Then he said he didn't have any homework. I talked to his teacher and knew that he did have homework. I also knew that he had just gotten a starter train set for Christmas so I told him that I would give him a new section of track (it cost 15 cents) for his set each time he did his homework. He began doing his homework. Then I stopped giving him the track and told him that I would get him an accessory every 2 weeks for the set if he kept doing his work. He did, and after a while, he and I just forgot about it and we spent our time doing other things together. But he's still doing his homework.

Of course, there had been some necessary groundwork before the Big and Little brothers began working together. The Big Brothers had undergone a 5-week orientation program at the clinic, in which the case history model was used as the primary teaching vehicle, combined with question and answer periods, general rap sessions and role playing of particular situations they might encounter. Sample situations were presented to them. For example, what do you do if you take the Little Brother to the basketball game, and he starts running around and does not sit in his seat? What do you do if a child misbehaves in front of you at his own home, and his mother is not at home? What do you do if mother disciplines the Little Brother in front of you? What should you do if mother starts telling you about her personal problems? After the initial orientation session was completed, the Big Brothers continued to meet weekly with the program director in group supervision. These weekly supervisory meetings consisted of lively discussions of individual cases, problems, and accomplishments. They also presented the opportunity for information seeking, feedback, and new ideas on approaches to the individual Little Brother.

Families of both Big and Little Brothers were interviewed before we started, and the program was fully explained to them. Curiously enough, the families of the Little Brothers did not show resentment when their child was assigned to a high school student rather than a mental health professional, and, in fact, they very quickly perceived that it might be a good idea. Families of the Big Brothers had to be reassured that their sons would not be dealing with "crazy" children who might be potentially violent. In addition, case assignments were made within limited geographic boundaries so that neither Big nor Little Brothers would have to cross wide expanses of alien gang turfs.

We began our program with only two Big and Little Brothers. Even with such a small number, it was difficult at first to get clinic personnel to refer Little Brothers to the program, because, after all, the Big Brothers were not the usual kind of therapists. However, soon the feeling changed to "we might as well refer them anyway since we have nothing else to offer them at this time," inasmuch as they were on the treatment waiting list. Now we have seven Big Brothers, five black and two Puerto Rican, and we have added two black Big Sisters. As the Brothers and Sisters proved to be successful therapists, the referrals increased.

The feedback from the schools and families of the involved Little Brothers has been almost uniformly very good. Although the program was not originally designed as a research project, there appears to be much in the way of face validity for it. The Little Brothers are doing much better in school, at home, and are no longer presenting the problems that originally brought them to the clinic. Rather a much more manageable problem of a different sort has emerged. The Big Brothers have been reluctant to discontinue their work with the Little Brothers after they improved, and they insist that a 10-hour a week experience of between 1 and 2 years is essential. The clinic director at one point suggested that perhaps they might work with two Little Brothers for only 5 hours per week, but the Big Brothers legitimately refused and insisted that they need at least 10 hours a week to really develop a firm relationship. The arguments around this point were of considerable resemblance to those of psychoanalysts when they discuss the need for an intensive long-term commitment to patients. The emphasis on the one-to-one relationship had been built into the program from the beginning as a way of both getting the Big Brother involved and in making his task less difficult than if he had to relate to many

children. It is probably a necessary phase in the early development of the
Big Brother, but in the future, we would hope that he could work with
several children. At any rate, it is clear that the Little Brothers have found
persons they can identify with, confide in, rely on, and trust.

As an unintended result, we found that the mothers of the Little
Brothers learned some different childrearing techniques by the intervention of the Big Brothers. Through observing the Big Brother in his
interaction with her child, mothers began to learn how to deal more effectively in areas of limit setting, consistency, as well as positive and negative
reinforcement. At the same time, they appeared to feel less threatened by
the Big Brother since he does not represent a formal mental health
professional who is telling them what to do. As informal observers of the
process, the mother gets some help in the shaping of her child's behavior,
but she is not placed in a role of a client or patient.

The Big Brothers themselves have grown considerably through this
experience. They have made valuable inputs into the overall design of the
program and have been very concerned about continuity once they
graduate from high school and leave. The "veteran" Big Brothers who
have been with the program beyond the first year participate in the
screening, selection, and orientation of the new brothers. Their own sense
of independence and personal identity has been strengthened through
serving as a role model and by having a child dependent on them. Our two
original Big Brothers, on their graduation from high school, went on to
college on scholarships. One is majoring in premedical studies with a
desire to go into child psychiatry, whereas the other is interested in clinical
psychology. These senior Brothers are also very active on their campus
and have hopes of initiating a similar program in their local community.
The identification process which was inherent in the program worked in
more than one direction through the Big Brothers modeling their career
choices on ours.

We, too, learned from them. Although their work is not yet central to
the work of the clinic, the Brothers have had a selective effect on our own
staff. Perhaps if they had functioned as cotherapists or junior therapists,
they would have had an even greater influence on staff who would then
have carried cases together with them. We wished to demonstrate,
however, that the Brothers' primary therapeutic efforts could in some
instances be comparable to those of the professional staff. We wished them
to be judged by their results as well as by their personal characteristics.
They did give us an excellent reminder of the fact that warmth, interest,
and dedication are just as important as sophisticated training and skills.
Once when we presented a review of the program to a budget committee of
the United Fund, one of the Brothers cut through the rather jargonistic

staff presentation and said, "Children are like puppies; if you're mean to them when they're little, they'll grow up mean. If you're nice to them and treat them right, they'll be OK when they grow up."

REFERENCES

1. Dept. of Health, Education, and Welfare, Office of Child Development, Research and Evaluation Division, Grant award guidelines, 1971
2. McCord J, McCord W, Thurber E: Some effects of paternal absence on male children. J Abnorm Soc Psychol 64:361–369, 1962
3. Biller H: Father absence and the personality of the male child. Dev Psychol 2:181–201, 1970
4. Santrock J: Paternal absence, sex typing, and identification. Dev Psychol 2:264–272, 1972
5. Wohlford P, Santrock J, Berger S, Lieberman D: Older brothers' influence on sex typed, aggressive, and dependent behavior in father absent children. Dev Psychol 4:124–134, 1971
6. Biller H: A note on father absence and masculine development in lower class negro and white boys. Child Dev 39:1003–1006, 1968
7. Cortes C, Fleming E: The effects of father absence on the adjustment of culturally disadvantaged boys. J Spec Educ 2:413–420, 1968
8. Mitchel D, Wilson W: Relationship of father absence to masculinity and popularity of delinquent boys. Psychol Rep 20:1173–1174, 1967
9. Herzog E, Sudia C: Fatherless homes: a review of research. Children 15:178–182, 1968
10. Herzog E, Lewis H: Children in poor families: myths and realities. Am J Orthopsychiatry 40:375–387, 1970

10

Mental Health Assistants

One brisk fall morning two black women left their offices at the Temple Community Mental Health Center. They were coworkers and friends, the dual relationship having grown through the hard years of training and experience as mental health assistants. As they walked to the bus, they talked of the morning's work ahead of them. Each was bringing her therapeutic activity into the real world of their clients: one to the home of a family, the other to the classroom of a young child. That act, repeated by these women and other mental health assistants thousands of times over the years at the mental health center represented three things: (1) the role of the paraprofessional mental health assistant as primary therapist; (2) the act of initiating an intervention into the life space of the client; (3) the fact that quality service can be made available to poor populations.

Corrina Caldwell, intent and determined, was making yet another of her countless visits to the Bellows family. An intact family, burdened with economic hardship, it was also a family whose members had paid a very high price to stay alive. The family had been referred to us from a pediatric outpatient clinic because of the serious problems presented by twins, age 3½, whose condition had been diagnosed as manifesting failure to thrive, secondary to emotional (maternal) deprivation. The pediatric program had worked hard and had used several resources in attempting to provide care for the twins, but they were unable to successfully gain the cooperation of Mr. and Mrs. Bellows. Thus, the family had a history of missed appointments, of suspicion and resistance to the efforts on the part of the clinic to work with Mrs. Bellows around meal planning, diet, and providing for emotional and psychological support for the children. The family had been referred to the mental health center with the recommendation that we direct our efforts toward helping Mr. and Mrs. Bellows reach the decision to place the twins in a foster home because of their apparent inability to provide adequate care for them.

After consultation with the referring agency, and after doing our own psychosocial, psychologic, and psychiatric evaluations, we reached the conclusion that Mr. and Mrs. Bellows' suspicion, distrust, and fear of outsiders which they used to protect themselves against the accusations of failure would defeat any intervention that was not based on the gradual development of a trusting relationship. This was the initial role of Corrina's work with the Bellows.

The twins, Tommy and Susan, were spindly, wan, passive children. Neither child had much functional speech. Their social repertoire was primitive. Their play behavior was stereotypic. And even their motor skills were underdeveloped for their age. Susan was somewhat more competent in terms of play behavior and sociability than Tommy. For both of them, however, food, affection, cognitive and social stimulation were all in short supply from their parents. Mrs. Bellows had lost the fight to apathy, passivity, and withdrawal. Mr. Bellows hammered at his wife verbally but could not act cooperatively. The organization of time and space in terms of eating, sleeping, bathing, and being together deteriorated into a rather amorphous unpredictable chaos. Food was hoarded and competed for. Members of the the family literally clung together in the home, having little outside activities but providing little emotional support or comfort to each other.

All of the five children languished, Susan and Tommy worst of all. All previous efforts by other agencies had been defeated by the Bellows' deep distrust, shame, and a battered sense of pride that could not admit final failure and could not give in to the ministrations of outside helpers.

After many visits and long and careful preparation, last week Corrina had been allowed to help Mrs. Bellows plan meals for the family. This simultaneously promoted improved nutrition and helped provide a basic structure to the family's day. Today, Corrina hoped to encourage Mrs. Bellows to spend some time playing and talking with the twins, one by one. Combining tenderness and persistence Corrina had worked cautiously with Mrs. Bellows, knowing that the woman's distrust and awful fear of failure stood between them. At the slightest feeling of threat, Mrs. Bellows withdrew, gave up, became silent, sullen, and psychologically evicted her guest. Six months later, after attempts too numerous to number, Corrina could see the visible results of her efforts. Tommy and Susan were in a Get Set Program. They had gained weight, were talking, active, curious children. Mrs. Bellows was in charge of herself and her children. The twins entered public school in a regular class. Now Mrs. Bellows' reluctance to have outside help was based on realistic self-reliance, but she could call Corrina when she felt the need for specific aid.

That same morning, Millie Thompson Bailey, tall and exuberant, was off to Balton School, to the first-grade classroom of her young friend Tina. Tina was one of two young girls in the same school who had manifested elective mutism. Tina had not uttered a word since school began. Her language had been established at the usual time, but in the past 2 years, Tina had only talked minimally at home.

Tina's teacher, frustrated and overwhelmed by a task she could not master, had at first been patient and cajoling, then angry and shrewish, and now had given up and in the main, ignored Tina.

Evaluations had been done, physical, psychologic, and psychiatric, and the diagnosis confirmed. Millie was the therapist working with Tina as well as her family. Into the room she breezed that morning, smiling a cheery greeting to the teacher, and then sitting down next to Tina. She had been trying several strategies. She had worked in the classroom with Tina alone and with another young classmate whom Tina had silently befriended. Using the usual school materials, Millie had used concrete rewards, first for gestural responses and written words, and then for even the slightest hint of verbal response from Tina. Millie had tried to use the relationship between Tina and her more verbal friend by talking with the other girl and hoping Tina's desire for attention and participation would loosen her tongue. Not only in class but on walks home from school and on visits to her home, Millie had worked in building a relationship with the frightened child. Smiles, nods, eyebrows, forehead, shoulder, hand and arm contact, all sorts of nonverbal business was transacted between the two of them, but Tina never broke her self-imposed silence.

The break came by an ingenious tactic that Millie serendipitously discovered one day. She had called Tina's home to inform her of a change in the time of her next visit. Tina, it was reported later by her mother, picked up the phone and smiled, recognizing Millie's voice. Mother noted that Tina started to respond verbally to the familiar voice but checked herself and then turned the phone over to her mother. When Tina's mother reported these events, Millie decided to add the telephone to her therapeutic tools. She would call and ask to speak to Tina and keep talking to her as long as the child held the phone. Finally, one evening it worked and through the earpiece came the faintest whispered hesitant, "Hello." Within weeks, the phone calls were real two-way conversations, and there was a spillover into face-to-face meetings. The first talking Tina did with Millie present was an analog of the phone. She whispered in her ear. From then on, the behavior generalized to whispered talk to Millie in school, then to other family members, in a much more expanded way than had previously occurred, then to children in her class, and finally to the much feared teacher. By the end of the semester, Tina was able to raise her hand, read aloud in a small group, and participate verbally both formally and socially in the school situation.

These vignettes represent two of many of children and families who have been directly treated and helped by the mental health assistants who had primary responsibility for care. In the past decade, the need for new sorts of manpower and new approaches to the employment of this manpower have generated a specific and growing response—the creation of "new professionals" or "paraprofessionals." The idea and its time had arrived. The subject of paraprofessionals in health and other service programs has been explored extensively by several authors.[1–5] As with any new practice, critics have questioned the usefulness and adequacy of paraprofessional training programs as well as the underlying concept itself.[6–8]

This chapter is not another theoretical justification or critique of paraprofessionalism, either in its notion or practice. Nor are we going to review in significant detail the origin and development of the mental health assistant training program at Temple Community Mental Health Center, since it has aptly been described by its originators.[9] We will discuss various questions about the practical issues of implementing a new paraprofessional program in a service institution. In this particular case, it was the employment of paraprofessionals in the Children and Family Unit of the Temple Community Mental Health Center. We will also examine the effect of the mental health assistant program and personnel on the structure and function of the mental health center. We will make several inferences, usually judicious but occasionally extravagant, to other types of mental health service programs.

First, let us summarize the Temple Mental Health Assistant Program by asking; Who are the mental health assistants? How were they selected and trained? Mental health assistants are a group of men and women, predominantly women, between the ages of 25 and 60. Most are black, although a few Spanish-speaking and several white persons have been in the two officially trained groups. The two groups were selected and trained in successive years, 1966–1967 and 1967–1968. After training the second group, a decision was made to wait a year before recruiting another group, with the intervening year to be spent revising and evaluating curriculum and training methods as well as the specific posttraining tasks the mental health assistant performed. Subsequently, training grant funds were not available and a new group was not formally trained.

Recruitment of the first two groups occurred through a variety of channels, including newspaper ads, radio announcements, contacts with local community groups, and by word of mouth. Members of the paraprofessional planning and training committee did the initial screening. This committee had begun working on the design for a paraprofessional program from the earliest days of the planning phase of the mental health center.

Applicants for the training program were screened by three staff members who rated them independently on several dimensions. The consensus rating or positive rating of two of three raters was required to hire. From the first group, 40 individuals were selected to carry out a census-like survey of a sample of the population of the catchment area. The survey was an end in itself since the administration of the center was interested in determining the characteristics of a representative sample of the population approximately 5 years after the 1960 census. This survey also served as a method of training and further screening of the interviewers, a subsample of whom would be chosen to enter the more formal training program and subsequently become mental health assistants. All members of the group chosen for this survey knew the entire plan at the time of their initial interview. Each was aware that of those chosen to do the survey, only some would be moved on into the mental health assistant training program. All of the interviewers were, of course, paid for that phase of the job.

The more formal training aspect of the program began after the population survey had been completed. Of the original 40 survey interviewers, 25 were chosen for the training phase. The training included several areas of subject matter as well as various pedagogical approaches. The curriculum included concepts of mental health and illness, normal and abnormal behavior, epidemiology of mental disturbances, methods of diagnosis and treatment, as well as the prognosis for various disorders.

The staff of the Children and Family Unit prepared a series of lectures, demonstrations, and discussions on child growth and development, child and family dynamics, diagnostic and treatment techniques used with children and families, and the uses and limitations of psychological tests.

The economics and practical aspects of mental health care as they applied to urban living, race, class and social institutions were also topics for discussion and presentation. Teaching methods included lectures, role playing, extensive demonstrations, and practice in interview technique. There were sessions on group identity building, as well as ventilation, confrontation, and sensitivity sessions. A special program was devoted to instruction and practice in self-expression, verbally and in writing. This was done since most of the mental health assistants' formal educational background ended at high school. Since high school, the trainees had worked in a variety of jobs as clerks, domestics, housewives, teaching assistants, and nursing aides.

SHOULD PARAPROFESSIONALS BE USED AS SERVICE PROVIDERS?

One of the first questions that can be raised about paraprofessionals is why have them in significant service roles at all? Prior to having put paraprofessionals in significant service roles in the mental health center, there were certain theoretical reasons for wanting to involve them in our program. After paraprofessionals had been trained and became active staff members, we learned some more realistic and significant reasons for their participation in mental health services. The first and preeminent reason to include paraprofessionals on our staff relates to the belief described in the chapter on the organization of the Children and Family Unit. We believed that many persons had latent or already developed skills in being helpful to children and families and that such talent and skills were not the exclusive domain of professional training or practice. A second and closely related reason is the necessity occasioned by the shortage of service personnel in the mental health field. The third reason is a two-edged sword without a handle. Standard formulation of this reason is that indigenous community workers are better able to relate to persons in poor communities than white middle class (or even minority middle class) professionals. Another way of putting this reason is that indigenous workers know the people better, have shared their experience, and hence know their needs and can communicate more effectively with poor, minority group clients. Further, we believed that the client will be more comfortable with the paraprofessional community worker than with the white middle class professional. Implicit or explicit in such class-based comments is a racial justification. Black clients do not trust white professionals; black paraprofessionals can communicate and work more effectively with black clients.

Support for this justification comes from the liberal, progressive professionals and from those spokesmen of poor and minority communities who have identified quite cogently the colonial status of many institutions in their communities. In urban areas, a variety of black groups have emphasized the development of a black consciousness and black identity among black citizens with the concomitant recognition of the pernicious effects of racism, psychosocial and economic, on both blacks and whites. Representatives of Spanish-speaking and American Indian populations express a similar viewpoint.

There is further justification, frequently not mentioned, but quite important. This is the argument concerning the economic impact of a newly developed mental health center or other service institutions in poor communities. A mental health center has an economic effect on any community, and thus bears an economic responsibility like any institution to the local population in which it resides and for whom it provides service. Part of this economic responsibility can be discharged by preferential hiring practices as well as preferential buying and purchasing of goods and services from merchants in the local area. Hiring practice particularly in positions beyond clerical and secretarial level brings new people into the service system in new roles. In the best and most reasonably planned approach, career ladders beyond the entry level are developed for the new careers or for the paraprofessional service giver even before he is hired. The above rationale belongs to the side of the aforementioned blade labeled "Use liberally against reactionaries, traditionalists, bigots, racists, and elitists."

There is another edge of that blade which can cut the wielder of the above argument. This hazard can be recognized and felt when someone raises the issue in the following way. Are indigenous paraprofessionals to be employed only in areas of poverty or with racial minorities? Is it just another form of second-class care with the crucial issue of distribution of professionals remaining untouched? Could it be that white middle class or other middle class professionals have devised and appropriately sanctified a moralistic way of turning over the "dirty work" to the "natives" while the colonials are protected and praised? Why is it that white and other ethnic and racial middle class professionals do not have to learn to talk, relate, appreciate the lifestyle of, deal with and serve the people who live in poor areas or belong to minority groups? Is it not possible that such a position as the one described in the first instance justifying paraprofessionals only counters elitism with elitism? As we lift our bloody hands from the edge of that blade, we see that it is labeled: "Specifically designed for puffery, trumpery, and pecksniffianism." There are no neat verbal or behavioral gymnastics which will avoid such a dilemma. The answers are in the doing.

WHAT SORT OF TRAINING FOR WHAT SORT OF JOB?

At this point, we will not discuss the broad philosophical and educational issues involved in training for professionals and paraprofessionals. Instead, we will make some specific recommendations for the training of paraprofessionals and the relationship of that to professional training and practice. To lay one myth to rest, the paraprofessional *is* interested in theory. She is interested in the "why" behind behavior. The best approach to transmit theory is one commonly used in all professional training, that is, case-oriented training emerging from and directed toward practical issues. Some comments about the transmission of theory on the part of professionals are in order. The professional who teaches and works with paraprofessionals had best be ready to shed his use of jargon for the nakedness of common words. Nakedness is embarassing and liberating at the same time. According to those who know about sexual mysteries, nakedness also promotes intimacy. What applies to the body applies doubly for the mind. If we recall the old fable, it was the clothes, not the emperor that were invisible. Making ourselves vulnerable in any relationship invites and challenges the same possibility in another. This is particularly true and important in the professional-paraprofessional relationship.

If the major task of the paraprofessional is to be a generalist and a primary therapist, then training should reflect the transmission and elicitation of clinical skills. If the agency adheres to a particular therapeutic mold or approach, then those should be the skills taught. If the paraprofessional is to be an expediter, case manager, or action-oriented environmentalist, other approaches are needed. For instance, is the paraprofessional expected to help do something about the child's school? Or help the family do something about their living situation? Or help a group of families who are concerned about recreation or housing? Such work is primarily intended to help local community groups develop their skills, capacities, and influence to deal with specific issues such as housing blight, drug traffic, and citizen-police relationships. If these are the skills to be developed and the task to be performed by the paraprofessional, then the training required should be based on the theory and practice developed out of community organization and planning.

There is a moral to be found here. Most mental health professionals have little training in consultation techniques, and very little knowledge about community organization. Therefore, it is illogical to believe that training paraprofessionals by psychiatrists and psychologists would adequately prepare them to become expediters or community organizational specialists. What is irrational in our approach at times is that we want the paraprofessional to be an almost godlike generalist, and we train them using personnel from narrow areas of professional specialization. Different sorts of training are needed for different tasks using different sorts of trainers. Clear ideas in the mind of the trainer about the tasks of the future paraprofessional result in sound training. When a training program is ill-conceived, poorly planned, and sloppily executed, it is an unmistakable malignant sign of the ambivalence, if not outright negativism, toward paraprofessionals on the part of professionals. Classism and racism can subtly appear in the psychological set of professionals. It is not overt, blatant bigotry, but the attitudes and behaviors that treat minority group coworkers as if they were not worthy of the very best effort, talent, knowledge, and skills that the professional has to offer. This is classism. This is racism. This is death to any kind of program, but more important, it is death to significant human relationships with coworkers. At Temple, the mental health assistants were trained to be generalists, but primarily clinicians. Some later trainees were assigned to the Consultation and Education Unit where their initial clinical training was of limited practical value.

WHERE SHOULD TRAINING TAKE PLACE AND UNDER WHOSE AUSPICES?

Should each paraprofessional group be trained by its sponsoring agency for its own specific tasks and uses within that agency? This develops a plethora of apprenticeship-type programs. Alternately, should training be carried out under the auspices of primarily educational institutions with field placement and hiring being done by various service institutions as the primary stage is completed? An important issue confronting the training of paraprofessionals is the issue of certification. Certification of training implies that there is some recognition across agencies, and even localities, of the quality and standards of the training program and of the competence and skills of the certified person.

The arguments against certification are those which contend that the usual institutions of higher learning have failed in the task of training humanly sensitive professionals. There is no reason to believe that the same institutions will do any better with paraprofessionals. One of the major crises in educational institutions today is the crisis of mechanical bureaucratic dehumanizing procedures versus an increasing concern for personalism and humanistic practices. There is some validity in the argument which states that professional training trains out the individualistic, spontaneous reactions necessary in being an effective helping person. This is another variant of the old head versus heart dialectic, one of the many similarly shaped bones that Western man has gnawed on for centuries.

Another argument against formal training and certification by educational institutions is that our society is obsessed with credentials, and yet it is the person, not the paper, that determines how well a human service task is performed. Such an argument is usually used by the credentialed or very lucky, very gifted noncredentialed. It offers little solace to the aspiring person who is beginning his training or seeking a career as a paraprofessional. To advise such a person that turning his back on credentials will bring about a change in social institutions or job hiring practices of agencies is to lie. We agree that too much has been made of credentials. To ask someone else to cut his own economic throat for the good of society, however, is not the solution and is hardly a clear sign of great human sensitivity and empathy on the part of the advice giver. However, should industry, service institutions, educational institutions, and legally established state certifying boards cooperate to alter the exaggerated role of credentials and provide the appropriate legal, administrative, and economic alternatives, then surely a new day will have dawned. It is to this end that certain professionals, both individually and organizationally, might work. This end is much more difficult to achieve, requires more time and effort, and essentially involves basic changes in the structure of our technocratic society.

Barring this sort of fundamental change, the prospective paraprofessional should find training in an accredited institution. If, however, on-the-job training is offered in the service agency which will then hire the paraprofessional, this agency should have connections so that the training can be recognized and certified by an accredited educational institution. Distinct advantages accrue, in terms of job mobility, better pay, and sharing with other jobs the usual channels of preparation and entry. Once hired, there are two additional features which determine the kinds of tasks and responsibilities of the paraprofessional. One, already mentioned, is the kind and amount of on-the-job training and staff development provided. The second feature is the quality, amount, and approach to supervision of the paraprofessional.

Some paraprofessionals come to the job with a bachelor's degree in psychology, sociology, or one of the newer mental health worker degrees or certificates. For others, as with the mental health assistants at Temple, formal education may have ended at high school, with some later business or vocational training. In this case, much of the training in mental health concepts and practice is on-the-job training in one form or another. Whatever the amount of prejob education, once employed the critical issue is the nature and the kind of supervision provided to the paraprofessional.

HOW SHOULD THE PARAPROFESSIONAL BE SUPERVISED?

First, let us dispose of rhetoric. Issues of class and race are everywhere. When supervision of minority paraprofessionals is discussed, one hears some of the same statements that were presented regarding service. Such statements can be made by professionals and paraprofessionals, middle class, lower class, black, white, and Spanish-speaking. These statements often run in the following vein. White middle class professionals are not able to adequately or effectively supervise black or other minority paraprofessionals. As a derivitive assertion of an ideology, such a statement has ideological uses. As a universal dictum or guide to practical action in the operation of a mental health center, such a statement is rhetoric. Let us for a moment dust off the old logical instruments. Some middle class professionals are unable to supervise some minority group paraprofessionals. Some white middle class professionals are unable to supervise anyone. Some minority group paraprofessionals had difficulty accepting supervision from white middle class professionals. Some minority group paraprofessionals had difficulty accepting supervision from any professional. Some paraprofessionals of any class or color and some professionals of any class or color have difficulty doing business together around supervisory issues under any circumstances. Having completed exercise one of Clear Thinking 101, let us proceed to deal with the issue of supervision. All paraprofessionals whom we have had occasion to work with seek, need, and expect high-quality, useful supervision. Such an attitude reflects the respect they have for themselves and the quality of work they wish to do. It also reflects the respect and concern they have for clients. No one wants to appear to self or others as incompetent. Mastery, that is, "being good at something," is a crucial part of effective psychological development and performance. To restate a basic administrative rule, mentioned in a previous chapter: If the online staff, individually or as a group, are not performing well, then the first place to direct repair efforts is at the supervisory level.

From the outset at Temple, much of the emphasis was placed on selecting and training of the mental health assistants with very little emphasis on the selection and *training* of supervisors. In fact, there was no adequate center-wide training program for supervisors. This is not unique, but common to most service settings. A professional, after some indeterminate number of years of experience, or after assuming a certain administrative role is deemed ready to supervise. Frequently, this occurs merely by administrative advancement within the agency rather than by demonstrated skill or talent. Finding, training, and supporting good supervisors is rarely an explicit program or function of mental health or any other service agency.

WHAT ARE THE CHARACTERISTICS OF SUPERVISORS AND THE SUPERVISORY PROCESS FOR PARAPROFESSIONALS?

The usual list of decent human traits apply here. In addition, the supervisor should be capable of clear, precise thinking and expression. The supervisor should be able to discuss material without using jargon, should not be heavily dependent on "process-type" notes. This latter requirement is a favorite mode of supervision directed at social work trainees. Particularly for those paraprofessionals whose writing skills are limited, this approach is arduous and nonproductive.

If the intent is to improve writing skills as part of the training of paraprofessionals, then such activities should be directed toward making clear, sharp, clinical observations and translating them into written statements. Such an approach is useful and needs as a supervisor someone who knows as much about making good observations and writing well as he does about mental health dynamics and technique. Helping a paraprofessional to divine the key content of an interview and commit it to paper in the most economic manner can be a very helpful part of supervision. This approach develops observational, perceptual, inferential, and writing skills.

The supervisor should be comfortable and skilled in using the onsite interview of the child or family as a basic vehicle for supervision. It can be accomplished in several ways: by having everyone in the interviewing room together, by using a two-way mirror, or by using a videotape. Audiotape, because of the degree of background interference, is a poor substitute. Exclusive reliance on verbal report from the supervisee to the supervisor is totally inadequate for anything but intermittent use. A supervisor should put himself on the line by demonstrating his own skills and techniques, responding to questions and criticisms raised by the paraprofessional. In turn, the supervisor must spend the time to observe, question, and criticize the paraprofessional in action. This reiterates the important theme of putting oneself on the line if one expects others to do it.

A next consideration is the way in which the onsite interview is used in supervision. If you observe an interview that I conduct, then there are two major approaches we can take in discussing that interview. One approach is to concentrate on my client: his appearance, behavior, responses, ways of expressing feelings, dealing with conflict and stress. The other approach is to concentrate on me, the interviewer: my goals and the strategies and tactics I used to reach my goals. You should examine my behavior, the kinds of questions and ways I phrase them, my responses and follow-ups to the patient's statements, the way I use bodily activity—all become part of the discussion. It is important that the supervisor have the ability to use both approaches. Particularly, the supervisor should have the ability to reflect on, discuss, and consider the techniques, goals, and methods that he, as interviewer, uses for different clients and different situations. Further, the supervisor should be able to do the same things with the paraprofessional supervisees. In the process of selecting supervisors, it is important that the administrator or head of the training program determine by actual observation how the potential supervisors can use various approaches to supervision. Another requirement for the supervisory relationship with paraprofessionals is the ability of the supervisor to identify and build on the particular strengths and interests of the supervisee. It is especially important to label these explicitly for the supervisee so that he or she recognizes the strength and can begin to consciously develop it. If, for instance, a paraprofessional is extremely good at active modeling behavior to mothers regarding dealing with their children, this should be pointed out. "I like the way you got up and walked over and took Johnny by the hand, removed the block he was about to throw and led him over to his chair. Then you reminded him of his task of drawing a picture of a man. You sat down, you pointed out to Johnny's mother what you did and why. That was a very effective demonstration and a very good way of teaching her and helping her." Another example is the paraprofessional who has developed or uses naturally active listening techniques. When this occurs, the supervisor should comment on it explicitly, using concrete examples from an observed interview.

If the agency promotes outreach as a major task of the paraprofessionals, then there had better be some demonstration home visits, school visits, and agency visits by the professional supervisor. It is wishful thinking to think that the paraprofessional without any training experience can find his way effectively through the bureaucratic maze of schools and welfare agencies, and automatically know how to use which channels of communication in establishing working relationships with a caseworker, counselor, or teacher. Teaching such skills by modeling and by apprenticeship is mandatory. The supervisor's ability to recognize, label, and make explicit his or her own mistakes in interviews, home visits, play sessions, or agency interactions is central to any of these modeling demonstration techniques.

Because the paraprofessional, like many novice professionals, attributes omniscience and omnipotence to the professional and supervisory staff, it is important to dispel these attitudes early by the frank, open and nonobsessive discussion of the supervisor's own limitations, mistakes, and failures. Such a skill on the part of the supervisors takes a high degree of self-awareness, reflection, openness, and courage. Certain persons can learn it, but it is not inherent in acquiring a certain degree, title, or sitting behind a certain desk. Someone, somewhere, must take the responsibility for instructing, helping, and supporting supervisors to do their task well.

IMPORTANT QUESTIONS RAISED IN SUPERVISION OF PARAPROFESSIONALS

One of the fundamental attitudes several of the mental health assistants at Temple expressed was doubt about their right to question clients about private, personal feeling-laden areas. They identified with the client in terms of background and experience and felt that asking personal questions was being nosy. They expressed the feeling that the client might not only resent the paraprofessional's questions but fear that the paraprofessional might gossip about him. The client might know that they are not professionals, and therefore not give them the trust, respect, or confidence of telling them about significant, difficult, or personal problems.

The paraprofessionals also had doubts about their own qualities or abilities to help people with their problems. Closely connected with this was the feeling that their personal lives were not problem free. If they were not psychological paragons, they were in that respect and to that degree hindered from helping others. If their own marriage was in trouble or had failed, how could they presume to help someone else in marital trouble. This issue touches the interface between the role of helper of others with personal problems and the fact that all helpers have personal problems of their own, both intrapsychically and interpersonally.

One way of handling this particular issue is to emphasize the positive side. That the mental health assistant has experienced a number of problems in living or psychological reactions of anxiety, depression, distrust, helplessness, and rage make it possible for her to identify and understand what a client may be going through. That the mental health assistant failed to satisfactorily solve all her problems and may still be experiencing some problems can add to her patience, empathy, and willingness to endure with the client in his or her particular struggle. Each of these doubts is related to the combined issues of paraprofessional status and the degree of experience in the helping process. Novices in the professions express many of the same feelings and attitudes, but these novices have several years of education and training to inculcate the requisite knowledge as well as the self-concept as a professional that justifies and rationalizes curious questioning and helps develop the skill of separating private distress from public performance. For the paraprofessional, the time span is much shorter. For the mental health assistants, the time from being selected to be a survey interviewer to finishing the training program and beginning on the job work as a clinical worker was approximately 9 months. Further, the knowledge that the paraprofessional has in terms of theory and practice is less extensive than that of the professional trainee. The marked difference further differentiating the paraprofessional from the professional is the matter of social sanction. The paraprofessional movement at this time has only limited social sanction from the larger society. The degrees of M.D., Ph.D., M.S.W., Ed.D., and even B.A. are not only statements of educational qualifications, they are a sign of society's green light. They summate a whole range of permissible and expected behaviors. Those same behaviors if performed without the aegis of these signs could result in everything from social criticism to legal action. Initially, the paraprofessional without a degree requires a great deal of external support to carry out those tasks which she fears she should not or can not do.

In our experience the often expressed concern on the part of professionals that paraprofessionals would take on tasks beyond their competence or would "get in over their heads" is not a serious risk. It is the other side of the coin, the hesitancy, lack of sureness, and exaggeration of limitations, personal or in terms of social sanction, that hinder the paraprofessional from fulfilling her full potential.

Paraprofessionals are eager to achieve quick results. This was a pleasant contrast with the expectations of most professional mental health workers that quick results are to be avoided and are suspect. One psychological source of this problem for paraprofessionals is the equating of commitment with effectiveness. There is a tendency on the part of the inexperienced and those who are uninformed as to the mechanical workings of service institutions to believe that the full and total solution to the problem of human service is an adequate quantity of individual and collective concern. Suspicion or derogation of technique and antiintellectualism, subtle or blatant, are frequent corollaries of this belief. Connected with the expectation of quick results is the belief in the magic of words. This belief is demonstrated in the reflex resort to exhortation and admonition in dealing with clients. This represents a common sense, rationalistically based approach to influencing human behavior. It clearly is useful and successful at times. Successful exhortation depends on the induction or elicitation of fervor and self-determination in the client, at times accompanied by the helper's enhancing mild degrees of guilt in the client. Frequently, such an approach does not succeed. It is particularly useless with those clients whose anxiety, guilt, or depressive affect markedly constricts or determines their attitudes or behavior. Children have been subject to a barrage of exhortation and admonishment from parents, teachers, principals, siblings, police, and ministers. Laying on more of the same will likely have the same effects as previous efforts and will confirm in the child's mind that the present helper belongs with the other adults who are out to prove the child bad or wrong. When exhortation failed, the mental health assistant frequently felt disappointed, questioned her own competence, and began to express the opinion that the client did not want or could not use help.

The supervisor's strategy at this point must be direct and explicit. First, the supervisor should be supportive of the paraprofessional's feelings and help her identify these, and the reasons for them. Then, the supervisor must deal with the central issue. Invoking basically unfamiliar and abstract theoretical concepts to help in clarifying this problem is of no use. Rather, the discussion should focus on the supervisor using her own personal or professional experience or asking the paraprofessional to reflect on his or her experience. An example is as follows:

> You know, we sometimes forget that when we respond to a person's problem with a lot of advice or you should's or why don't you's or if you hadn't done that, we're just repeating what the clients have told themselves or what others have already told them many times. If they have not been able to follow such advice until now, it is doubtful we will be successful. Just think of your own experience when you've had a problem. When other people just tell you what is best or what you should do, they really don't take into account the feelings involved or the difficulties you or I might have had in carrying out what we already know we should do in that situation.

Another way of putting this approach is to draw on the supervisor's own experience.

> I find whenever I feel frustrated or become irritated with a client or a client seems stupid or cruel that I end up preaching at them. In one way or another, I let the client know I disapprove of them or imply that I am somewhat better because I can tell them what to do.

Such an approach, if it is truthful and not mere artifice accomplishes several things. It provides an identification of supervisor and supervisee in terms of fallibility and feeling. It also provides the same sort of modeling of openness to one's own negative feelings which can be labeled and discussed without shame or guilt.

Another important technique in the supervision of paraprofessionals is to help them identify a manageable or definable problem and establish some definable goals to accomplish. This approach can be discussed within a theoretical framework. We used the notion of the therapeutic contract. Using this concept, we suggested that the mental health assistant and the parent or child would work out an agreement regarding what problems they would work on, how, when, and in what way they would try to work together. For children who are preadolescent, this approach requires modification so that it is cognitively manageable. For the child younger than 6 years who is to be the object of direct treatment, play techniques are used and discussion of the therapeutic contract is limited to particular immediate agreements around activities within the therapeutic hour.

As a general rule, the mental health assistants as well as the professionals within the Children and Family Unit did not do much therapy with children below the age of 7. Invoking our principle of parsimony, we encouraged most of this work to take place through the relationship developed by the helping person with the parent.

Within the supervisory relationship, a good deal of work was directed at helping the mental health assistant deal with the understandable ambivalence she had toward parents or children. With young children, the hazard to avoid was that of being critical or judgmental of mothers and fathers. With the adolescent, the risk was identifying with the parental role from their own personal experience and reacting negatively to the sullenness, antagonism, and disturbing behavior of the adolescent.

In establishing definable goals and a working contract, we emphasized helping the client gain control over some area of life and becoming more of an initiator of action rather than merely a passive respondent to the vagaries of fate or the initiation of others. We promoted this approach in terms of encouraging alteration of internal processes, feelings, and thoughts, as well as promoting altered kinds of behaviors in dealing with other persons or conditions. Throughout all this, we stressed the importance of understanding the stage of the relationship between client and therapist, and how the therapist herself could be the initiator of effective action in using the relationship to help the client reach their agreed on goals.

With children, the approach was modified according to age. We believed the mental health asistant should become a real and tangible person in the child's life. We emphasized joint interviews of child and parent as well as individual interviews. The mental health assistant elicited feelings from the child, served as a broker or moderator between child and parent, or child and school personnel. The mental health assistant made direct suggestions of alternate ways a child might express his feelings or deal with troublesome classmates. We suggested that the mental health assistant use positive reinforcement with the child or parents. We also instructed the mental health assistant to guide parents in using relevant, specific, positive reinforcement in dealing with problems presented by their children.

We used the same approach in our supervision. After a short training period, the mental health assistants were thrust into a significant helping role. Initially, the mental health assistants were uncertain and lacked self-confidence in dealing with a variety of issues. Faced with such a situation, it is natural for all of us to hear criticism and amplify it, leading to overreaction in one way or another. The criticism then could be heard by the mental health assistant in stereotypic terms: professional versus nonprofessional, white versus black, and authority versus subordinate. It is around such issues that the human qualities as well as the training and supervision of the supervisors become the critical factor. If the supervisors personally and in their roles are able to identify such reactions in the paraprofessionals as well as in themselves, they can then initiate open, direct discussion that diffuses the exaggerated reaction to criticism and enhances the confidence of the paraprofessional. This promotes the kind of working relationship between supervisor and supervisee that can be used as a source of strength and development for both.

REFERENCES

1. Sobey F: The Nonprofessional Revolution in Mental Health. New York, Columbia Univ Press, 1970
2. Reiff R, Riessmann F: The indigenous nonprofessional: a strategy of change in community action and community mental health programs. Community Ment Health J Monograph No. 1, 1965
3. Pearl A, Reissmann F: New Careers for the Poor. New York, Free Press, 1965
4. Rioch MJ, Elkes C, Flint AA, Usdansky BS, Newman RG, Silber E: National Institute of Mental Health pilot study in training mental health counselors. Am J Orthopsychiatry 33:678-689, 1963
5. Klein, WL: The training of human service aides. In Cowen EL, Gardner EA, Zax M (eds): Emergent Approaches to Mental Health Problems. New York, Appleton, 1967, pp 144-161
6. Steisel IM, Adamson WC: The use and training of allied mental health workers in child guidance clinics. J Am Acad Child Psychiatry(in press)
7. Steisel IM: Paraprofessionals—questions from a traditionalist. Prof Psychol 3:331-342, 1972
8. Cooper S: Role diffusion—dilemmas and problems. In Gottesfeld H (ed): Critical Issues in Community Mental Health. New York, Behavioral Publications, 1972, pp 235-260
9. Lynch M, Gardner EA, Felzer SB: The role of indigenous personnel as clinic therapists: training and implication for new careers. Arch Gen Psychiatry 19:428-434, 1968

11

The Incentive Specialist Program

In a previous chapter, we have described patterns of consultation between schools and mental health agencies, with particular emphasis on the pitfalls which may occur. In this chapter we examine, in considerable detail, the development, implementation, and maintenance of one specific consultative venture—a positive mental health intervention at the junior high school level. This program represented a joint effort between the Children and Family Unit of the Temple Community Mental Health Center and the Young Great Society, a black community self-help group developed in Philadelphia in the midsixties.

THE PROBLEM

Poor children have a high risk for dropping out of school.[1] Poor children who are in school have a high probability of manifesting some form of educational retardation: reading two or more grades below level, scoring low on standardized tests, and showing signs of perceptual motor dysfunction. These same children have a high risk for developing attitudinal, motivational, and behavioral manifestations of maladaptation in school settings, including apathy, restlessness, disruption, boredom, depression, a sense of futility, and most eroding to self-esteem, a sense of

Special acknowledgments are warranted: Dave Berger, for his research leadership; Don Bruce, for his direction of the Specialists; Althris Shirdan, for coordinating the research activities; Skip Gump and Ted Blunt, for their roles in the initiation of the program.

failure and incompetence.[2-7] Poor urban, black children have a high risk for all these disabilities. The remote or initial etiologic factors are the subject of study and hot debate.[8-11] Concurrent etiology or maintenance causality is another issue. We directed our intervention more directly to the latter issue.

OUR PHILOSOPHY

As we have indicated, the Children and Family Unit of the Temple Community Mental Health Center was responsible for developing consultative and intervention programs with schools and other community agencies which have primary responsibility for children. In the theoretical approach of our unit we emphasized positive mental health intervention. We believed in finding ways to identify and promote strengths, skills, and abilities in persons or in groups with whom we consulted or intervened. This is in contrast to those approaches in which attempts are made to identify and work with children who are manifesting disturbance, emotional disorder, or other kinds of handicaps.

We had the twofold intent of increasing the self-esteem and confidence of both our clients and our consultees so that they would be more competent in their daily life activities. We wished to promote the useful, effective, and satisfying functioning of the person or group in the particular social setting in which he or they operated. For children, this consists primarily of three spheres: family, school, and friends. To be able to live in some harmony in day-to-day relationships with family members, to work effectively in schools so as to become a competent learner, and to be able to relate on a mutual basis with peers, constitutes what we chose to call "making it."

Our main focus in consultative intervention was to enhance the skills and ability of primary caregivers and social agents to help children "make it." In schools, we were interested in helping teachers, counselors, and other school personnel in their direct work with children. A number of similar strategies are presented in "Emergent Approaches to Mental Health Problems," edited by Cowen, Gardner, and Zax.[12]

We also believed that some of the difficulties found in schools could be attributed to the mutual alienation of the school as an institution from the population it was responsible for serving. We, along with many others, felt that this was a particularly cogent factor in schools attended by poor, urban, minority populations.[13-15]

One useful role of a mental health program for children would be to attempt to promote ways in which this mutual alienation could be diminished. A tangible effect of this approach would then be to help children "make it" in schools. We set out to make such an attempt.

EARLY PROGRAM

The Young Great Society is a community self-help organization started in West Philadelphia in 1966 by its founders, Herman Wrice and Andrew Jenkins, as an effort to deal positively with gang violence. Over the years, the organization has grown and diversified, established neighborhood community centers, a health clinic, a moving company for poor families, a housing rehabilitation program, an overnight youth hostel, and an economic development corporation.

The relationship between the mental health center and the Young Great Society had a fortuitous beginning in late spring 1968. The vice-president of the Young Great Society, who later became the director of the Incentive Specialist Program, sought help for a community resident at the community mental health center. In the process of providing help for this client, the director of the Children and Family Unit learned of the history of the YGS, and specifically of a YGS program that had been in effect in summer school the year before in several West Philadelphia elementary and junior high schools. In addition, the vice-president of the YGS had previous experience teaching in a junior high school in North Philadelphia.

As an outcome of these early discussions, the staff of the Children and Family Unit and the YGS organized seminars for teachers in a local school in the summer of 1968. These particular teachers were recent graduates and new teachers to the Philadelphia School System. The principal of the school had encouraged the joint approach that the mental health center and the YGS offered. The YGS emphasized the community issues of urban living, including aspects of race, poverty, poor housing, poor health care, lack of employment, and the multiple ways in which the social institutions affect the lives of the poor and black people. The mental health center staff discussed such issues as psychological growth and development, psychosocial conditions for effective learning, and problems that inhibit effective learning. We also discussed aspects of communication, both verbal and nonverbal, reviewed the uses and abuses of psychological tests, described the availability of mental health services in the community, and the method by which clients could obtain those services. In addition, we described ways in which such mental health services are abused by schools using the extrusion process when they deal with problem children.

During the summer, we had joint YGS-mental health center meetings to plan for the development of a fall program in one of the local junior high schools. This latter program evolved into the fully developed Incentive Specialist Program which persisted in the same junior high school for 5 years.

CHOICE OF POPULATION

Seventh graders were chosen as the target population. They are at pubertal age and experiencing all of the physiologic and psychosocial changes accompanying this critical phase of development. Socially, they are moving from the top rung of elementary school to the bottom rung of junior high school. The curriculum, rostering, departmental structure, and overall size and complexity of the junior high school are modeled after the senior high school. This, in itself, along with the pubertal issues, makes seventh grade a period of potentially high stress.

Though feeling the early stirrings of independence, the junior high school student is still very tied to adults. We felt that the support of a relationship with a young adult, who is neither parent, teacher, nor older sibling could be helpful to the emerging adolescent.

ROLE OF THE INCENTIVE SPECIALIST

As described above, the fundamental purpose of the Incentive Specialist Program was to promote more effective adaptation of children to school and to enhance their school performance. Several methods were used to reach this goal. The central strategy was to place young, black adult community paraprofessionals called *incentive specialists*, in selected classrooms. They were to work with all the children in that classroom. Their efforts were directed particularly to those children who were experiencing difficulties in effective learning, in terms of motivation, behavior, and accomplishment. In addition, the incentive specialist worked to promote better relationships among students in these classes, and between the students and their teachers. The specialists also attempted to mobilize the parents' educational concerns and interests by informing them of their children's activities, accomplishments, and problems in school. The specialist tried to elicit the parents' active involvement in helping their children to learn at home as well as promoting contact between parents and school personnel.

What are the tasks that the specialists were initially expected to perform? In addition to the central and crucial task of establishing effective relationships with teacher and students as described above, the specialists were expected to perform some specific tasks in the classroom contingent on the agreement between the specialist and the teacher.

1. They were to work as clarifiers, explainers, for any and all children in a class to help increase understanding of the day-to-day instructions,

lessons, and homework assignments. To accomplish this, they needed to work closely with the teacher and to understand and participate in the teacher's lesson plans. They particularly helped those students who were not doing well. They explained assignments, helped students organize their work, and tutored individual students or groups who were identified as needing assistance with a particular assignment.

2. They were to promote, wherever possible, students helping each other so that students would involve themselves in a somewhat different role in the classroom rather than the usual one of being a passive listener or learning merely for himself. The student would also be learning so that he could, on occasion and when he felt competent and comfortable, help another student. The specialists were encouraged to help each student give to each other, as well as receive help from each other. It was part of the specialist's role to facilitate and make possible this kind of give and take.

3. The incentive specialists hoped to open up a three-way teaching process so that it was not just limited to students learning from older people, but that teacher and specialist could listen to and learn from students. The specialist served as a resource and feedback person to the teacher. The specialist informed the teacher about how the material was being received and comprehended by the students. As he came to know the students well, the specialist was in a position of suggesting alternate ways of relating the material to the students. The specialist's own life experience, and his understanding and involvement in the lives of the students, was used in offering suggestions for engaging the students in the learning process. Through his relationship with the incentive specialist, whose background was somewhat similar to that of the student, the middle class white or black teacher might learn how to get closer to his classroom students.

EXTRACURRICULAR ACTIVITIES

First, the specialists were required to visit the home of each student in their respective classes. The purpose of the initial visit was to acquaint the parent with the incentive specialist program, to introduce the specialist to the parent, and to discuss any possible concerns, problems, or questions the parent might have about the program or about his own child's educational difficulties. Selected follow-up home visits were made for those children with whom the specialist was working intensely, and in which additional parental involvement was important. At times, home visits were made at the request of the teacher or the counselor for the purpose of transmitting to parents some concerns or questions school personnel had about a particular student.

Second, the specialist conducted field trips with small groups and classes of students. These field trips were combined education, social, and recreational events. They were to enhance the students' knowledge and experience in the larger world outside of the school and particularly that aspect of the world in which black adults were involved in significant activities: cultural, athletic, educational, and vocational. Individual specialists who had talents, skills, or interests in a particular area would work after school, in the school building, with groups of students who shared an interest in this activity. Such programs included athletics, gymnastics, charm school, beauty culture, fashion design, and less formal, but significant, involvement in some of the larger community activities of the YGS in North Philadelphia.

Third, specialists also initiated and organized several major school functions which involved large numbers of students beyond the particular classes with which they were working. In the first year, they promoted a ninth grade prom, which students and faculty attended. The specialists organized assemblies in which students, specialists, and other invited guests participated. These included outside speakers as well as musical and entertainment groups. In the final year of the program, the director of the YGS wrote, produced, and directed a hard-hitting play centering on the issue of drug abuse, highlighting its individual, social, and racial aspects. This play was not only performed in the involved schools but also in several other schools for an audience of students, faculty, administrators, and general public. In addition, the play was taped by one of the television networks for local use.[16]

ADMINISTRATIVE PERSONNEL

The director of the Incentive Specialists, who was the YGS vice president, had overall responsibility for the recruiting, interviewing, and selection procedures for the specialists. He was also responsible for the major part of the training of the specialists in preparation for their tasks. He held regular meetings with the specialists, including training and problem-solving sessions. He dealt with day-to-day problems that arose in the school concerning the program, and was available to the specialists for advice, consultation, and support. At times, he served as mediator between the individual specialist and the faculty or administration. Together with the project director, he maintained close liaison with the involved teachers and administrators.

The overall director of the project was a child psychiatrist, who was the director of the Children and Family Unit of the Temple Community Mental Health Center. He had administrative responsibility for the project both in its intervention and research aspects. During the first two years, a member of the Children and Family Unit staff served as a project coordinator. This person carried the day-to-day ongoing coordination of the overall project with the director of the Incentive Specialists. He also spent time working with the specialists on group techniques, group dynamics, and the important psychosocial factors at work in the classroom and school among specialists, students, and teachers. In the latter years of the project, many of these duties reverted to the project director.

The project director was responsible for the initial and ongoing negotiations, as well as for the continuous review, planning, and coordination of the program with school administrators. He participated in specific activities regarding the teaching and training of the incentive specialists, particularly as these related to the psychological development of adolescents, intrapsychic and interpersonal dynamics, family structure and dynamics, and the interactional and social dynamics of the school and classroom. In addition, he provided individual sessions of a supportive nature to specialists having a crisis or problem around their work.

The psychiatrist attended many of the regular meetings with the teachers, counselors, and specialists. His participation added more structure to the meeting and increased the verbalization of teachers. In a mental health capacity he provided consultation regarding particular children to incentive specialists and school personnel. On some occasions, with parental permission, he provided consultative evaluation of children in the school setting. Other children and their families were referred from the psychiatrist, school personnel, or incentive specialists to the mental health center where evaluations and direct services were carried out.

TRAINING OF THE SPECIALISTS

During the summer preceding their entrance into the classrooms, the incentive specialists underwent an intensive period of training. They met daily with the director of the Specialist Program, who provided background information on the Young Great Society and described how the Incentive Specialist Program had originally developed. Role playing was used, including simulation of a typical school situation with teachers, students, counselors, and families. Basic information about the seventh grade curriculum was presented, including the various topics that the children were expected to master. Problems in learning and tutorial approaches were discussed. The psychiatrist and a psychologist from the Children and Family Unit provided in-depth material on pertinent psychological and social matters, as already described.

Meetings between the specialists and their director emphasized black awareness and identity. There was also consideration of what kinds of trips and experience could be planned that would enhance the children's knowledge and experience of the larger society, especially those areas in which blacks played a major and significant role. In addition, readings were assigned in areas of education, black literature, adolescence, and social and urban problems. Beyond the summer preparatory period, the same kinds of teaching activities were carried out on a less frequent basis throughout the school year, immediately after school and on Friday afternoons. These were supplemented by case or problem-centered discussions that revolved around a teacher or child. Later meetings were also held with the whole intervention staff who discussed issues such as conflict with teachers, problems in role definition and territorial threat, professional putdowns, teachers' anxiety about children's behavior, and concerns about specialists' and teachers' effectiveness. Such methods as long, uninterrupted lectures, dictation directly from books or notes, and copying out of books were considered very negative and ineffective methods used by teachers. Ways were discussed in which teachers might "hear" suggestions about other approaches that the specialists might offer or model.

RESEARCH DESIGN

After the incentive specialist program had been effectively installed in one junior high school, we decided to expand it to two schools and to carry out an evaluation of the program. The School District of Philadelphia contributed funds for the expansion, and a National Institute of Mental Health Research Grant awarded in 1970 supported a 2-year evaluation of our intervention.

Our expanded intervention program, now complemented by the research design, was conducted in two junior high schools within the catchment area. Incentive specialists were assigned to three classrooms of seventh graders of each school. Each classroom had 35 to 38 students. There were, therefore, about 110 seventh graders enrolled in the active or intervention group of the program in each school. An additional three seventh grades were identified in each school to serve as the comparison or control group. These children were not directly exposed to the active work on the incentive specialists.

A number of measures, both objective and attitudinal, were used to determine the impact of the specialists. We obtained children's grades in subject, attitude, and behavior, as routinely reported four times a year, in addition to a measurement of the children's achievement on standard tests. We collected behavioral information on a number of children who were given discipline slips or suspended. We obtained data on children's attendance, the number of children who moved out of the school and out of our program, or into the school and into the program. We also had information on the contacts of children with counselors, and on any children who were referred to the mental health center for services. We collected information regarding staff absences, staff turnover, and the frequency and distribution of substitute teachers. Information was collected concerning the specialists' visits to students' homes.

We developed two instruments for measuring attitude which were administered to children and staff of the school. The first instrument was the Children's Attitude Toward School or CATS, and the second, the Staff's Attitude Toward Schools or SATS. Each of the instruments had approximately 110 items, 15 items common to each scale.*

IMPLEMENTATION OF THE PROGRAM

An applicable paradigm, at least for the beginning of the program, is that of salesmanship. We were selling a set of ideas, beliefs, and skills and the way to apply them. We had a conviction that this "software" will make things better for children in schools. The children are the tenants, but we have to convince the landlords. The landlords have to be convinced that the program will be beneficial to the children and not harmful to them. It is critical and often not made explicit by the landlords that they must be convinced that any program will not upset the delicate balance among staff, teachers, administrators, counselors, and others.

At the early stages of the beginning of our incentive specialist program, we had not really clearly conceptualized the notions of overt and covert consumers (see glossary Table 1.1.). In the instance of the school, children are the overt consumers and staff are the covert consumers. Children consume knowledge and the time and effort of the staff. The staff consumes money, status, power, and perquisites. As these latter are always

---

*Children's Attitude Toward School and Staff Attitude Toward School were developed by D. Berger, A. Shirdan, D. Bruce, and W. Hetznecker. These two instruments were designed to assess children and staff attitudes toward school. After directions were given, the CATS was administered to an entire class. Each item was read aloud. A single response to each item was recorded on a four-point scale representing degrees of agreement or disagreement.

differentially distributed in any institution, there is always maneuvering to gain the most advantageous position as determined by the priorities and values of the individual person and those of the institution itself.

Specifically, it is "better" to teach a class of bright children than slow learners. It is "better" not to need help, advice, or guidance in teaching than to "have to depend on" others such as aides, curriculum specialists, and administrators. Teaching English, math, science, or social science is "better" than teaching gym, home economics, art, or shop. Teaching is "harder" and therefore "better" than counseling. Alternatively, counseling deals with the "problems," and therefore is "harder" and "better" than teaching. It is "better" to have a "quiet" class by whatever means that to risk being disapproved of by peers or principal for not being able to "control" the class. This is an extension of the formula: If you do not have control, you cannot teach.

Mental health workers are trained to be aware of and take into account the importance of feelings in determining behavior. We are well aware that anxiety, hostility, and feelings of inadequacy, guilt, frustration, and depression can significantly affect how people adapt. Further, we know how to apply these ideas to consulting or intervention programs in terms of the consultee.[17-19] Then, if we are concerned about those feelings, we must be prepared to deal with them.

Two questions to ask in designing a program before one starts the initial negotiation is as follows: "Is my program directed primarily toward overt or covert consumers? If what I am proposing is good for the children, that is, the overt consumers, how could it be bad for the staff, the covert consumers?"

Well, then how to begin? How in this case means with whom. In any institution or system there are "no" sayers, and there are "yes" and "no" sayers (Weiss' Law).* Many people can say "no," a small number can say "yes" and "no." Thus, there are always more people in any institution or situation who can stop or hurt you rather than help you. The following vignette is given by way of illustration:

Tommy calls Jimmy on the phone.

Tommy: Can you come over and play, Jim?

*Weiss' law was first enunciated by E. Weiss to W. Hetznecker on the latter's induction into the maze of Washington bureaucracy. The law states that in any organization there are people who can say "no" and there are those who can say "yes" and "no." The kinds of possible responses are a function of role or position not of personal whim. There are always many more "no" sayers than "yes" sayers in any organization. The probability of finding a "yes" sayer increases as you go up the hierarchy. The last statement needs the qualification that territorial control is often as important as simple rank in the hierarchy of the organization as to whether one has the "yes" saying power.

Jim: I have to ask my mother. Mother, can I go over to Tommy's?

Sam (Jim's older brother):   Mother is at the store and she left me in
                              charge.

Jim: Sam, can I go over to Tom's and play?

Sam: No, I can't let you.·You'll have to wait until mother comes home
        and ask her.

This is the "yes" and "no" function at work in the family system.
Sam can say "no," mother can say "yes" and "no." This basic structure
applies in more complicated systems. "Yes" and "no" are functions of
position, role, and office. A teacher could not say "yes" or "no" to a
program being introduced at the school level, and in fact, would not even
be asked until the program directly affected her classroom activities. If
that same teacher is appointed vice principal or is elected union
representative for all teachers in that school, she suddenly acquires a "yes"
and "no" function of some degree. However, it is important to remember
that same teacher did have a "yes" and "no" function relative to her
students and because of some territorial rights had·a "yes" and "no" capacity in response to certain directives of the principal.

When dealing with individual teachers or administrators, it is important for mental health workers to avoid reductionism, which frequently
·amounts to looking at the world through id-colored glasses. Simple decla-
rations of "she's for the program" or "she's hostile" or "she's passive-
aggressive" are inadequate. They are parochial and formulistic ways of
trying to account for the response of someone by using an in-group dialect.
Such an approach may be reassuring but is a totally inadequate explanation of social phenomena.

Personal qualities, intrapsychic conflicts, and personal styles do affect
how people conceive of and carry out their social roles. But "good guys"
and "bad guys" are also made by reason of being behind a certain desk or
bearing a certain title. The vice principal for discipline is a "bad guy" until
proved otherwise from the students' perspective. It is an absolute necessity
for those who are selling a program to a system to understand in some detail the limits and range of "yes" and "no" saying inherent in any job in a
system.

We identified at least two major "yes-no" people: the district
superintendent and the principals of those schools in which we wanted to
work. Now, how do you talk to the first? The answer is "yes." Here is·a
specific example of "ham and eggs," the double-contingency paradigm.
(See glossary, Table 1.1.) If the superintendent says "yes," it will help us

gain the principal's agreement; and the superintendent is more likely to agree if we already have the principal's agreement. One solution, then, is to approach both "yes" and "no" sayers at the same time. One could suggest a joint meeting of superintendent and principal to discuss the proposal. The hazard to this approach is that everyone's public face and image are on the line. Such a meeting can turn into a vehicle for carrying on preexisting struggles or conflicts between certain parties in the meeting. These conflicts will probably have nothing substantially to do with the mental health workers or their program. In the process, they can become the scapegoat victims in a power struggle. Such a meeting can be diagnostically helpful, just as a joint family interview can demonstrate crucial interactions. However, one must assess the possibility of good and bad results of such a tactic.

The other approach is to see each "yes" and "no" sayer independently for purposes of informing each of the central aspects of the program. In such a meeting, one can transmit specific information regarding the program, respond to questions, with the goal that the "yes" and "no" sayer will review the description of the program and consider meeting again. One then aims for an agreement to consider undertaking real negotiations regarding the program. It is very important to present a written proposal at the time of the initial meeting or immediately afterward for the parties to read, consider, and respond to at the next meeting.

At this point, that is, at the next meeting serious negotiation begins. An initial proposal should be a short, concise, clear statement of the purposes of the program, the personnel to be involved, the sort of approval or commitment that is being requested of the school, who the specific persons are and what procedures will be involved for both the school and mental health staff. Some estimate of duration and possible cost should be included. If financial support is to be sought from the school or sources other than the sponsoring mental health agency, this should be stated.

Every bargain or deal is based on a quid pro quo. The school is looking for some clear statements or criteria by which they can estimate what they are getting for what they are giving. The more concrete, specific, and operational a mental health program description or proposal can be, the greater the likelihood is that it will gain a fair hearing from schools or other service institutions. It is important to remember that mental health workers are selling snake oil (see glossary, Table 1.1) and not buttonhooks or pencil sharpeners. Even though the specific ingredients of the snake oil are difficult to specify, it is our responsibility to say how we will apply it, on or with whom, what it will cost, and what the expected tangible results are.

TRAFFIC CONTROL

Sherlock Holmes referred to the significance of the dog which didn't do anything in the night. The questions you do not ask and the "yes" and "no" people you do not know you have to see can hurt you. To paraphrase another old slogan, "Ignorance of a system is no excuse." You still pay the price.

One example touches on the research aspect of our incentive specialist program. We had made it clear to superintendents, principals, and other administrators in the school system that our program was to be a combined service and research program. The research aspects had been discussed in some detail in the written protocol we had circulated to various school personnel. We had submitted a National Institute of Mental Health research grant application in which we indicated that we had school district approval, which we believed we did have. We were about ready to start the program when an administrative assistant in the local superintendent's office said rather casually one day, "I don't see any letter of approval from the research office of the school district approving your research plan," and we said, "What research office? What sort of approval? No one told us." And he, smiling the Cheshire Cat smile of a helpful bureaucrat, replied "Oh, of course, any research program has to have approval from downtown. The director of research has to approve the scientific merits of the study as well as being assured that the rights of children and teachers are not infringed upon." We in one chorus responded, "So how do we get that approval? Whom do we see? How long does it take? This was midsummer, about a month before school was to begin. We wanted to start the program the first week of school, having completed all the administrative preparation ahead of time. After much flurry and fury, after submitting letters and protocols, and after several meetings, we acquired the requisite approval. However, this delayed us about 6 weeks in initiating our program. The moral of the fable is find a map and a trustworthy guide to lead you through the maze of bureaucracy.

Never assume anything. After reviewing our project proposal the district superintendent approved it and even agreed to provide a substantial amount of seed money to be used for part of the specialist's salary in each of two schools. We were overjoyed. This would allow us to start the program early in the year and would be helpful in our efforts to obtain money from the federal government since it was evidence of the school's commitment to the project.

A few weeks later we met with the newly appointed principal of one junior high school in which we wanted to continue the program from the previous year. He was understandably cautious about supporting a program begun by his predecessor. As we discussed the funding of the program by the district, it became clear to our surprise and embarrassment that the money that the superintendent had promised us was the money that the principal had been counting on to employ additional staff. He was angry and felt betrayed. It was exactly the kind of situation in which a power struggle could have developed at the expense of our program. As a result of the reasonableness and fairness of the principal he chose to handle the situation in a manner in which our program did not become a casualty.

IMPLANTATION

Any system views outsiders with suspicion. This is a given response. The degree and type of response varies with how close the outside threat becomes. The consultant visiting once weekly to meet with teachers or counselors or to sit in briefly in a classroom might generate some anxiety and defensive maneuvers. But a program such as the incentive specialists in which outsiders are introduced into the inner circles of the institution causes a reaction very similar to the foreign-body reaction in the human body. The reaction of the school personnel was compounded because the incentive specialists were paraprofessionals, and were not directly employed by the school.

People in schools already have stiff necks from the over-the-shoulder syndrome, each group looking back over their shoulders to see who on the next rung of the peck order is checking on them. Introducing the incentive specialist just fixes the neck in a permenent torticollis position.

What sort of response did we get to the program after its initial introduction to the school? This varied from school to school and from class to class, but there are basic similarities. Some of the responses can be listed as follows:

1.   How come our school was picked?
2.   Do you think our kids are worse off than kids in other schools?
3.   It's that same old trick—white folks doing research on black kids.
4.   We don't need any research. We don't need any help.
5.   What qualifications do they (the incentive specialists) possess for work in schools?
6.   What are they going to do?
7.   What if we don't want an incentive specialist in our class?

8. They aren't going to tell me how to teach.
9. How will you know if the program is effective?
10. Are you just trying to prove black kids are crazy and need mental health?

These are the initial kinds of questions that occurred in one form or another throughout the early stages of the program. They also recur at the beginning of each new school year when the program is reintroduced, even though it had been in the school for a year. Although some of the teachers, principals, and program members are the same and are known to each other, the same concerns surface and must be responded to with respect and understanding.

Having obtained the agreement of the superintendent, we turned to the task of explaining the project to the faculty and counselors. It is all well and good and absolutely necessary to get the principal's agreement before anything can begin, but unless one has the support, agreement, and active cooperation of the teachers, the program is in for difficult times and probably ultimate failure.

The initial task of explaining and introducing the program to the staff of the school should not be left to the principal alone. Since the principal is the administrator, he is accustomed to sponsoring something, explaining it, and then instituting it as rapidly as possible. When introducing a program such as the incentive specialists into the school, one must have the principal's support and backing, but also much more. The principal should introduce the intervention team at a faculty meeting, and then have the team describe the program and respond to questions. A brief written description, highlighting the essentials of the program, should be available to faculty. It is also important for the intervention team to remain after the meeting to field questions and be accessible to the teachers in subsequent weeks for teacher discussions about the program. Much to our sorrow, we did not implement such a complete initial approach during the first 2 years of the program, but after some unfortunate experiences, we did begin to follow this procedure in later years, with the result that the faculty was more cooperative.

Following the initial introductory meeting, we then had a series of small group meetings with teachers from different grade levels and departments. We began to narrow down and focus our efforts on building a speaking and then a working relationship with teachers of the active and control classes in the seventh grade.

It is important to assert from the outset that initial agreement, initial understanding, and initial pledges of support are no guarantees for ongoing understanding, support, and cooperation. Defensiveness, resistance, hostility, confusion, apathy, indifference, and concerns over territoriality, status, and class and race issues are not dealt with once and for all. Such issues are constantly emerging and constantly have to be handled.

MAINTENANCE AND REPAIR FUNCTIONS

Maintenance and repair operations in an ongoing program, even one which last only 1 school year, are crucial. They are not often written about and not planned carefully in advance. Usually problems are dealt with on a day-to-day, crisis-to-crisis basis. Maintenance and repair are really part of administration and are part of the administrative role of each member of a program such as ours, with varying degrees of responsibility. The time devoted to maintenance and repair may vary according to the level of responsibility, but each member of a program needs to know, to recognize, and to identify those aspects of the program that require constant maintenance and repair. In addition, the intervention group must share strategies and problem-solving techniques that attend to this significant aspect of the program.

As we have described, when a new or an outside program comes in contact with, or is placed in a host institution, reactions and interactions, on the part of the host and the new program are many and variable. One analogical and somewhat oversimplified way of viewing it is in terms of the response of a host organism to the grafting of a replacement organ. Such examples are common today and include transplants of hearts and kidneys, and the most common of all, replacements of blood. When grafting an organ, the surgeon is most interested in matching the degree of compatibility as close as possible. Such is the reason for transplanting kidneys from one twin to another, one sibling to another, or one member of a family to another. An assumption is made that there is greater genetic and basic tissue similarity between the donor and the recipient in such instances. After transplantation, the major concern is that the host may reject the organ. Many techniques and procedures have been devised and are still being researched to reduce, eliminate, or modify the rejection response so that the grafted organ might "take."

In looking at the interactional field of a new program in a host institution, one can look at some of the same forces at work. There are two major contrasting forces involved in such an outside "grafted" program. One force is the force of extrusion and rejection. In one way or another, the host institution devises means to get rid of the new program completely. Failing to accomplish complete rejection, the host institution, in this case the school, attempts to devise ways of making a program less threatening or less noxious. Such approaches tend to trivialize the importance of the program, diminish its functions, and diffuse its operations by modifying the roles or tasks of the personnel. For example, in one class, the incentive specialists were exclusively used to hand out papers, to xerox materials, and to sit in the back of the room in a sergeant-at-arms or policeman function. Another approach is to sideline the program. This approach effectively removes the program from the central function of an institution, to a sideline position. For instance, an attempt was made to use incentive specialists as nonteaching assistants to monitor lunchroom activities, rather than as colleagues in the teaching process.

The other major force that works on a program is the process of engulfment, assimilation, and incorporation. In this operation, which frequently begins at the time of the early negotiation with the administration, the host institution attempts to take over control of the operations of the new program in the school. It wishes to be totally responsible for defining all roles and activities, and to control all the movements of the specialists. In addition, the host starts to view and to use the specialist in ways that are familiar and traditional for paraprofessionals to be used in schools. Thus, they become essentially a group of nonteaching assistants, classroom aides, or people who work in the office, helping secretaries with such matters as dealing with absenteeism, late slips, or medical excuses.

Another more subtle method of assimilation occurs by means of the interpersonal relationship between a specialist and a staff member of the school. We believe strongly that the quality of interpersonal relationships among specialist, faculty, administration, and counselors determines if a program such as ours is to succeed. However, that very relationship can be used at times to co-opt, intentionally or unintentionally, the specialist and the program. This can be accomplished by taking advantage of the sense of isolation, of being a stranger or an intruder in the school that the specialist experiences not only in the initial stage but recurrently throughout his work in the program. The assimilation occurs as the specialist is encouraged to form an essentially school-related identity in which he sees his primary allegiance and loyalty to the school an an institution. He begins to assume roles that are essentially identified with and determined by the school. This shift accomplishes two ends: it relieves the specialists's anxiety and his feelings of isolation, loneliness and differentness, and at the same time it brings him closer to school personnel and enhances his feelings of belonging and acceptance.

There are no easy and pat solutions to dealing with either one of these major processes: extrusion and assimilation. However, they must be identified, recognized, and planned for in advance. One method of preparation is the use of anticipatory guidance given to specialists. It was of paramount importance to help the specialist with his anxiety and feeling of isolation. On the part of supervisory staff of the program it is important to take the initiative to provide formal and informal support to those on the firing line. When a program fails on the firing line, the first place to look for difficulty is in the relationship of supervisors to line workers and in the failure of the administrative personnel to attend assiduously to the maintenance and repair operation.

To illustrate further the need for maintenance and repair functions, we must make some distinctions among those aspects of an institution which are essential, central, or permanent. A lunch program is central but may not be permanent. Counseling in many schools is permanent, but its centrality varies from school to school, city to city, and time to time. Reading as well as math and gym will always be taught in the school. The special Behavioral Research Laboratory Reading Program which was contracted by the school district to produce certain results within a certain time will not necessarily be back again the next year. Dropping the BRL program or a particular approach to math or science is one thing. Dropping reading or math altogether or cutting severely into their time allotment is something else again. Eliminating reading is not a possible consideration in the school today if it is to retain an essential characteristic of its identity.

However, the incentive specialist program is not in this status or position at all. It is an "extra," a "trial," or a "could be eliminated any time" program.

The methods of maintaining essential, permanent, or central function or program are built into the structure of the program. In the school, the table of organization, the allotment of time and space, the assignment to classes, the purchasing of materials, the organization of committees or departments, the flow of memoranda, and the regular meetings and contacts between staff and administration are all part of the maintenance and repair function.

An outside or expendable program is not an integral part, and does not automatically enjoy the benefits, of the repair and maintenance processes that operate on central functions. To maintain a program like the incentive specialist program or any other newly begun or newly introduced program, one has to look for other ways. In fact, one finds that a maintenance process which preserves and protects central functions of the school program may be acting in a way as to exclude, eliminate, or cripple newly implanted accessory, "nonessential" or "peripheral" programs.

A concrete example is in order. For an entire school semester, the incentive specialists had no space assigned for such functions as meetings with students to discuss problems, meetings among themselves, or meetings with a teacher or a small group of teachers. They did not even have space assigned to store their materials or to hang their coats. They used the faculty lounge, but found it totally impossible to meet there with students who needed their help. By definition, students were excluded from the faculty lounge except for specific purposes of serving the faculty, such as carrying messages or helping duplicate papers. In addition, the specialists experienced a perpetual state of discomfort because they had no desks of their own and constantly were having to give way to faculty who assumed a priority status over the use of equipment and resources. Socially, the specialists felt uncomfortable and were made to feel so because they were not faculty and technically did not belong there.

We spent hours of meeting time directed toward the acquisition of space for the specialists. The principal and all others were sympathetic. But space was, in fact, at a premium. Finally, the specialists were assigned a small 8' x 4' room which had served as a book storage room. It required several months before that decision could be reached. The final solution was a very significant one. The room maintained its original function as a book storage room. But a few bookshelves and some other miscellaneous material were removed so that the room could accommodate three or four chairs and a small table. Thus, the original *central* function was maintained and the incentive specialist was given only squatters rights.

Whatever commodity is in short supply will be jealously guarded by the owners in an institution and very grudgingly will any of the outsiders or tenants get any of these goodies. To provide the incentive specialists a clearly defined space of their own was to admit the possibility that the program could become permanent and could compete for centrality of position. A host institution or system will resist this notion very strongly. The resistance is not a "good guys"–"bad guys" phenomenon. This resistance is a manifestation of the complex psychosocial realities of institutional processes. At the affective level, the main threats in any social system are threats to status, power, approval, and the fundamental threat, that to survival.

We were aware of these threats, but we did not assess them carefully enough nor deal with them effectively until the second year of the program. The autonomy of the specialists, and their intentionally ambiguous role definition was very disturbing to the teachers. The hope and tactic was to encourage each teacher and specialist to negotiate a mutually satisfying relationship and definition of role task for that class and subject. If that approach foundered, the director of the specialists was to be consulted either by the specialist or teacher and hopefully the three parties could work out something. The group meeting of teachers and specialists together was intended to explore problems of working relationships and to provide an opportunity to discuss solutions that teachers and specialists had worked out. We had money allocated in the grant to pay teachers at the standard rate of pay for overtime activities. Initially, these meetings were too poorly attended by teachers to provide an effective vehicle for solving problems and dealing with the issues cited above. The specialists also had been too uncertain and too reluctant in inviting the teachers to the meetings and in pursuing them to obtain a committment for their participation. The teachers, on their part, were threatened by the meeting, sensing confrontation or a vehicle for criticism.

Both groups were quite defensive. The school as a social institution does not promote such discussion in its ongoing regular maintenance and repair activities. Therefore, this was a new vehicle and a new methodology for school personnel. In addition, the teachers did not feel that their input into such meetings would have any significant effect on defining the role or altering the task of the specialist. They were bothered by the vagueness and ambiguity of the specialist's role, and did not wish to, or did not feel comfortable enough to take the bull by the horns and work explicitly with the specialist to define mutually acceptable roles. Therefore, the general response was one of withdrawal, aloofness, and unwillingness to engage in discussion about the problems that the program engendered or the approaches to solutions.

By the second year, we had learned our lesson and had become much more explicit in defining the specific tasks we wanted the specialist to perform. We had previously obtained from the teachers throughout the year and at the end of the first year's experience suggestions on how to improve the program. These included some specific recommendations about what the specialist might be more useful in doing in the classroom. Such an approach was more acceptable to the teachers since they recognized that they had participated in and had some control in defining how the outsiders would work in their classrooms. Even though we had stressed this throughout the first year, and had attempted to use the day-to-day relationship between the specialist and teachers as well as teacher-specialist meetings for defining this relationship, the approach had not worked well. By the second year, some familiarity with the specialists as well as a feeling of being less threatened by the specialists helped the teachers become more active in a constructive way in dealing with the issues of maintenance and repair, especially those dealing with task orientation of the specialists. Teachers, in general, we should note, are much more comfortable in dealing with issues such as specific tasks and goals. For teachers, as for most individuals, discussing interpersonal relationships is very threatening, and it takes considerable support and practice for them to become not only comfortable but effective at it. Therefore, it seems a more appropriate initial tactic for outside programs to focus on such things as task-directed activities when meeting with groups of teachers. The problem with this approach, however, is that mental health workers on their part are less adept, less skillful, and less comfortable in employing such concrete task-oriented role-directed tactics. By the second year, the modified approach that we had taken reduced the ambiguity of uncertainty for both teachers and specialists, provided predictability and structure, and hence, reduced anxiety and defensiveness on both sides.

The most formidable threat to the maintenance of an outside program is the issue of competing priorities. Specifically, the members of the incentive specialist program, whether specialist, researcher, or mental health professional, needed to be aware that we were competing for attention, recognition, time, and space with well-established priorities that influence teachers, counselors, and administrators. For the goals of the program, it was a priority for the incentive specialist to meet with teachers regularly both in one-to-one and regularly scheduled group meetings, as described above. This was our priority, but clearly not that of the teachers in the early years of the program. The inducement of money helped elevate these meetings in the priority ranking of teachers but still not sufficiently to get a regular turnout of large numbers of teachers.

No doubt emotional factors acted as partial deterrents. But in addition to these salient factors which mental health people could detect and deal with, there were significant and realistic individual and group priorities which affected a teacher's decision not to attend meetings. Some teachers had to attend graduate school classes after school, and these classes were valued because of grades and credits which added to the teacher's status, pay level, and advancement in the school system. Some teachers needed to go home to children and families, or they had other personal committments. Some had second jobs. In each of these instances, the priorities were such that the meetings with the incentive specialists and other staff of the project came in second, third, or were not even in the running. Some teachers felt that they would gain nothing by such meetings anyway and thought that the program staff had nothing to offer them. This was at times a statement of status and caste mentality and at times an accurate appraisal of the usefulness of the meetings.

Those responsible for an intervention program must compete actively for a sacred time commitment from the principal on a monthly basis, at least. These meetings serve the review and planning functions (see Chapter 7). This time also represents an opportunity to obtain from the school administration any information about major changes in curriculum or other school matters which could affect the program. One of the major purposes of regular meetings is to achieve some degree of centrality for an outside program at a top level. Time is the most precious commodity, and it must be fought for. An agenda should be developed and both sides should contribute to it.

Another important strategy is to find allies within the system who can support the program and be available to inform the rest of the school staff of the program and its benefits. These allies also keep the program staff aware of complaints and problems that are not directly presented to them. We found counselors especially helpful in this regard. The particular tradeoffs for this alliance was case consultation by the psychiatrist and direct service from the mental health center when the counselor requested it. The counselors were helpful in providing information regarding the larger school issues, especially since many had been in the school longer than anyone in the program, and they were able to transmit something of the history and tradition of the school. Such a microhistory of an institution is invaluable in understanding the why's and wherefore's of the existence of certain procedures and role relationships.

Several informal friendly relationships between incentive specialists and teachers provided also review and feedback functions. The tradeoff expected of the incentive specialists is that they be willing and able and competent to pick up on problems presented by children in counseling or classroom situations. Teachers and counselors particularly began to use the specialists for home visits. Since the specialist viewed home visiting as part of his central role, he was quite eager and willing to accept this tak.

Finally, even after a partial "take," a "new" program is "new" several years running. Some of the initial negotiations and implantation activities must be repeated, almost replicated each August and September. The half-life of most school consultation-intervention programs is approximately 1 school year. Programs that survive and are renewed or reborn in the same school the second, third, or more years are exceptional. By this alone, they can count themselves successful. The price for this level of success is an inordinate amount of time and effort devoted to maintenance and repair.

REFERENCES

1. Report of the Joint Commission on Mental Health of Children. Crisis in child mental health: challenge for the 1970's. New York, Harper & Row, 1969
2. Coleman JS et al: Equality of Educational Opportunity. U.S. Dept. Health, Education, and Welfare, Office of Education. Washington, D.C., U.S. Govt. Printing Office, 1966

3. Golden M, Birns B, Bridger W, Moss A: Social class differentiation in cognitive development among black preschool children. Child Dev 42:37–45, 1971

4. John V: The intellectual development of slum children: some preliminary findings. Am J Orthopsychiatry 33:813–822, 1963

5. Whiteman M, Deutsch M: Social disadvantage as related to intellective and language development. In Deutsch, M, Katz I, Jensen A (eds): Social Class Race and Psychological Development, New York, Holt, 1968, pp 86–114

6. Rohwer WD: Learning, race, and school success. Rev Educ Res 41:191–210, 1971

7. Kappelman M, Luck E, Gantner R: Profile of the disadvantaged child with learning disorders. Am J Dis Child 121:371–379, 1971

8. Deutsch M: Happenings on the way back from the forum; social science, IQ, and race differences revisited. Harvard Educ Rev 39 (3): 523–557, 1969

9. Jensen A: How much can we boost IQ and scholastic achievement? Harvard Educ Rev. 39:1-23, 1969

10. Jenks C, Smith M, Acland H, Bane MJ, Cohen D, Gintis H, Heyns B, Michelson S: Inequality: A Reassessment of the Effect of Family and Schooling in America. New York, Basic Books, 1972

11. Kagan JS: Inadequate evidence and illogical conclusions. Harvard Educ Rev 39:274–277, 1969

12. Cowen E, Gardner E, Zax M (eds): Emergent Approaches to Mental Health Problems. New York, Appelton, 1967

13. Kohl H: Thirty-six Children. New York, New American Library, 1967

14. Dennison G: Lives of Children. New York, Random House, 1970

15. Hetznecker W, Bruce D: The role of a community mental health center as a mediator between school and community. Paper presented at annual meeting of American Psychiatric Association, Miami, Florida, 1969

16. Bruce D: Dope for Dummies, 1972

17. Caplan G: Theory and Practice of Mental Health Consultation. New York, Basic Books, 1970

18. U.S. Dept. Health, Education, and Welfare, National Institute of Mental Health. Mental Health Consultation to Programs for Children. McClung F, Stunden A: Washington, D.C., U.S. Govt. Printing Office, 1970.

19. Hetznecker W: Dimensions of Consultation, chapter in report to task force on school consultation of American Psychiatric Association, (in press).

Part IV

Overview

12

Review and Inquiry

We were recently privileged to obtain a historical memoir written by Frère Gilles of Beziers, a fourteenth century Dominican monk, while he was resting for a few weeks in the retreat house of St. Eulalia, in the south of France. A portion of the document includes a dialogue between Frère Gilles and Frère Auguste of Languedoc, a Dominican colleague who was also temporarily on retreat after a rather busy year as a mendicant preacher to the poor. Apparently, it was the custom of these two brothers to meet over a glass of wine before vespers and to discuss matters of theology which troubled them. One of their conversations, as recorded by Frère Gilles in his diary, follows:

Frère Auguste: I have been thinking about our previous conversation, Frère Gilles, and some questions still puzzle me. We speak about sin, how difficult it is to achieve grace, and yet, how can we as priests, prevent sin? Our numbers are so small, and we have so much to do.

Frère Gilles: Should we, or perhaps the better question is, can we prevent sin? I feel that such is an impossible task, for sin is all around us. Look at all the temptation man encounters. We can hardly expect him to remain without sin through our humble efforts.

Frère Auguste: Perhaps the Albigensians were right, despite the teachings of our learned colleague, Thomas Aquinas. Their belief that God, being responsible for all things, is also responsible for evil, is borne out by the ubiquity of sin. The times seem to breed sin. But if this is so, are you content with only helping those who have already sinned and continue to sin grievously, rather than strengthening our people to resist sinful thoughts and acts?

Frère Gilles: No, content is not the right word. Rather, I am skeptical. After all, look at the conflict which raged between the Albigensians and the Thomists around the question of the perfectability of man. This kind of argument, as well as other disputes within our church with which you are quite conversant, has been going on for a long time. There has been so much written about the causes of, and the conditions for, sin. We seem no further along in our understanding of it.

Frère Auguste: Yes, but sometimes such theological controversies mystify, rather than clarify. We all know sin when we see it. What is more difficult to detect is the presence of grace and holiness in another or even in ourselves.

Frère Gilles: Perhaps, but what about the different circumstances of sin, especially those internal and external events which limit man's knowledge and will. For example, is a poor man who steals bread as sinful as a rich man who cheats?

Frère Auguste: No. I think not. Holy Scripture instructs us to be charitable and to show mercy. If I may presume to quote, "It is easier for a camel to go through the eye of a needle than for a rich man to enter into the kingdom of God."[1]

Frère Gilles: Such quotations tend to make a virtue out of poverty. My Abbé is constantly reminding me that we must produce more butter, eggs, and wine for the market or we shan't have enough francs to see us through the winter. But I am straying from the point. Let me come back to your original question about sin, and whom we should help. If we are to use our offices to keep people from sinning, how can we do it? I agree with you, we are only a relatively small handful of priests in the midst of many sinners.

Frère Auguste: I suppose through our words, faith, and deeds. I know that the manuscripts can only be read by a few people, so we must rely on our preaching.

Frère Gilles:	Frère Gilbert has an interesting idea. Not a novel one, but he espouses it with great vigor. He insists that former peasants and those who have sinned most heavily make the best priests. They are the ones who have the greatest influence on the people, especially the poor.
Frère Auguste:	While his experience may differ from mine, I do not agree. The people wish to respect someone who is learned, someone who can reveal God's word, someone who can point the way to a better life through salvation.
Frère Gilles:	It is also a highly impractical idea. It would be quite difficult for peasants to become priests, at least in any great number. Further, can we expect knights, lords, and kings to pay any attention to the remonstrances of a former peasant now cleric?
Frère Auguste:	In such an event, the universities or seminaries would have to give courses in manners, as well. But I must confess, some of my teachers, while offering the best in philosophy and Latin, did not prepare me well for preaching, which is a rather worldly matter. When I actually began my work, there was much I did not know.
Frère Gilles:	In that respect I envy our Benedictine brethren. They rarely leave the monastery, and are free to pursue scholarly interests for years and years.
Frère Auguste:	Perhaps we can be grateful that we at least have had the opportunity during this retreat to discuss our concerns and to renew ourselves.
Frère Gilles:	Yes, these weeks of retreat are helpful. And now it is time for vespers. Let us go.

In reading this document, we had great empathy with these two clerics who were struggling with critical issues within their profession: how to define sin and grace, conceptual notions central to their work; how to assign degrees to sin; what to do first, and how to do it; how to teach others to do it; and who make the best priests (doers).

Using these two brothers as our inspiration, we too retreated, looked back on our endeavors and recorded our speculations about our own roles, tasks, and priorities. A typical religious retreat combines elements of three stages: recollection, confession, and resolution. After our own fashion, we sought to use the same technique. Possessing less wisdom than our historical counterparts, our conversation is perhaps more fanciful and less informed. Nevertheless, it reveals our impressions about our work and ourselves.

DAY ONE: ROLES AND TASKS

Marc: Now that we are in this isolated spot, insulated from our day-to-day worries, let's talk about some of the issues that concern us. First, I suggest we consider our roles and tasks and how we feel about them. Or, what are we doing anyway?

Bill: You know, one of the traditional ways to talk about the physician's role is that he is to treat, or heal, the sick and the ill. And, as we discussed in a previous section, that kind of medical model has its limitations. Another way to view things is to look at our social role in terms of what society's implicit and explicit expectations are. In that sense, the concept that Hughes uses of the "dirty workers" could be applied.[2] We are asked to be "dirty workers." Mental health workers of various sorts are supposed to take care of the casualties in the social process, that is, those who are troublesome or troubled. Usually, this means that they are sent to us, to our clinics or hospitals or institutions. That is our traditional role and no doubt some of the people sent to us do need our help. But another way of looking at this process is to see that a central task of mental health workers and the programs they develop, whether for children or adults is to prevent the process of extrusion. Troubled kids become troublesome kids and become sand in the gears. Every social system has its ejectors and rejectors. These are not bad, mean, child-hating persons, not at all. These are people who occupy certain social roles, uniforms if you will—desks, offices, titles—all of which add up to a simple function: get the troublemaker out of here. Such people can be school counselors, pediatricians, other psychiatrists, or ward staff. The extrusion can be partial or complete, temporary or permanent, and is frequently intermittent and recurrent. The family itself can extrude one of its members because the family can no longer cope with him, nor he with them.

Marc: Let me interrupt you at this point, if I can, or should I say if I may, and make sure that I am clear on what you are saying. Society has some basic faults and there are many people, including children, who are not getting what they need from the total human community or who just do not "fit" or adapt. Those of us in the helping professions, such as child psychiatry, are asked by society to be the "dirty workers" and to pick up the pieces. In that sense, we are in the same league with welfare workers, garbage collectors, and the police. Is that right?

Bill: Right.

Marc: Okay. But do you believe that some children need to be referred to mental health clinics? Do you believe that some need day care, special classes, hospitalization, residential treatment, group homes, or delinquency rehabilitation centers? Do you believe that some children should be removed or placed away from the noxious influences of family, peers, or neighborhood? Are you suggesting that we don't do that, even if it may be helpful to the individual child in certain circumstances?

Bill: Well, you know the answer is "kind of yes," but not for some of the reasons for which it is done: not as the first way of dealing with children who are troublesome in this way; not out of desperation, anger, retaliation, frustration, helplessness, or all the other myriad feelings that children generate in caregivers when the children aren't making it and, therefore, the caretakers aren't making it. Not until all the other reasonable resources and strategies involving people, time, space, and money have been tried by the folks in the mainstream, tried and found wanting. Not until steps 2, 3, and 4 that follow step 1 in the process of extrusion, have been thought about and planned for. It seems to me it is part of our job to help those who are the caretakers and who are struggling with these very difficult children to help them, if possible, find ways to continue to work with these children in the mainstream situation.

I say that as a statement of principle or belief. I also think it is important to add that, and I do not know how you feel about it, we as mental health workers have not learned how to best help teachers, parents, police, or other caretakers to really use their available resources or use other ways of helping these very difficult children. I have not stood in a classroom teaching 30 pupils, 3 or 4 of whom are really out of control. I know how much trouble I have maintaining order and control at my own dinner table, much less in a classroom, and therefore, I know that although the belief and principle are there, I am not sure I know enough about the technology nor am very successful in accomplishing it.

Marc: Basically, I agree with you. "Prevention" is certainly one of the favorite, "in-group," jargonistic words bandied about these days. Yet, we have very few tried and tested methods of prevention, even though we emphasize it. Prevention is a difficult concept to apply, especially since the mental health field cannot agree on a definition of illness. How can you prevent something if you are not sure what causes the problem you are trying to prevent? Prevention is a concept really borrowed from public health and epidemiology, and there are doubts about its applicability within the mental health field. Preventing an outbreak of cholera and preventing underachievement in school are similar conceptually only in that the word prevention is used in both instances.

And yet, I think we should support the notion of prevention, especially in terms of how one looks at a problem. For instance, when a family brings us "a difficult child," we should not take over as the expert, try to "cure" the child, and look at the whole encounter as if it is only between that particular child and us, as the therapist. Rather, it seems to me, our role is to help the parents and child deal more effectively with each other, to mediate the situation, even to, in a certain sense, translate their messages back and forth to each other, to clarify their behaviors for each other. We can shore up their positive resources, and in every way possible help them function as an integrated unit that no longer needs the help of an outsider to carry on.

Bill: Let me see if we can separate out two notions in our discussion, at least for my own clarification. We can't prevent a specific illness because we lack the knowledge of the factors and sequences of events which led up to the manifestation of the disturbance. Therefore, we don't know where or how to intervene. Prevention in that sense means increasing the probability of the non-occurrence of an illness. However, when I was talking about extrusion and preventing it, I was speaking about preventing a social process that occurs in response to the disturbance or distress manifested by a child in this case. It is that social process which says, "This child is sick, send him to the psychiatrist," or "This child is sick, get him out of this school," or "This child is disturbed, he should be in a special class or a hospital." That is the social process in which we have a preventive role.

Marc: And in terms of our beginning discussion about roles, I think what we are suggesting is that the child psychiatrist should really be an intruder into various social systems to help stop the process of extrusion, rather than serving as a "catcher in the rye" who rescues the recipients of the extrusion process. In a general sense, the child psychiatrist should be an educator of the extrusion agents, and many of the different kinds of people who work with children in their daily experience. So, hopefully, he will assist these others as they work with normal and unusual children, and will aid the involved social institutions in terms of changing their attitudes and belief systems about children. It is a somewhat overwhelming task, to say the least, but is reminiscent of the early child guidance movement in this country. For instance, Stevenson[3] felt that the clinic's role in education was more important that its treatment function, and in one of my favorite quotations, James Plant noted that each child referred to the clinic was "a random sample of community neglect."[4]

Bill: It seems to me that when you are saying "the child psychiatrist should," you are really making a statement about what we feel child psychiatrists should do in the future. Let's try to enlarge on that for a minute. If we have served as transitional child psychiatrists, moving out of one role and into another, what are some of the other tasks, aside from educating the caretakers, that should fall within the domain of the child psychiatrist in the future?

Marc: Well, getting back to a rather concrete clinical matter, the child psychiatrist must have greater involvement in the care and treatment of the "more sick" child, that is, the borderline psychotic child, the brain-damaged child, the child with sensory deficits, the multiply handicapped child, and the emotionally disdurbed child with severe medical problems. However, our past training has generally been in the area of treating the "less sick" or mildly neurotic child with adjustment problems. In the future, one might anticipate that these lesser difficulties will probably be handled by changes in the cultural socialization and adaptive processes. That is, as the special wisdom of psychiatry, psychoanalysis, and psychology become the property of the general public, parents, teachers, and other caretakers will become sensitized to appropriate ways of dealing with minor problems in children. It's what is "left over," that is, the "sicker" child, who should demand more of our attention.

Bill: There are other kinds of "sicker" children, or at least children who are at great risk for the development of severe psychosocial problems. These are the battered children, juvenile delinquents, children in welfare centers, children in residential and correctional facilities. Working with these children has not been personally or professionally attractive to the child psychiatrist. These children have been "losers." Yet it is ironic that the early history of child psychiatry shows that our discipline was very interested and involved in problems of social welfare.[5] For the past 30 years, however, our track record has not been very good and we have had very little input in this area.

Marc: We probably moved away from an involvement with juvenile delinquency specifically because results of treatment were quite discouraging. But our role may not be that of therapist, but rather as advocate and consultant, that is, to bring more of a psychosocially oriented perspective to those social institutions, for example, courts and departments of welfare that deal with these children.

Bill: Well, if we as child psychiatrists believe that children are affected by their environments, and if these are children who live in grossly inadequate environments, then we have an ethical responsibility to uphold our beliefs through our work. It is possible that if we do not accept this responsibility, society may impose it on us, at least on those of our membership whose work is supported by public and governmental funds. For instance, under Pennsylvania commitment procedures, implemented by the county mental health plan, some juvenile offenders are being directly committed to psychiatric hospitals whether or not the psychiatrist agrees, and psychiatrists are being subpoenaed to give testimony in a variety of juvenile court cases.

Marc: In contrast, one area likely to be a "winner," that is, attractive to the child psychiatrist, is the field of learning disability. We are frequently asked to evaluate a child who has a learning disability, and yet we have little training in the physiology of learning, the evaluation of children's cognitive and perceptual skills, or in educational and remedial planning. This whole subject is becoming increasingly popular both in general culture as well as in the specialty professions, and we have not been well prepared to be very useful, at least when things move beyond the emotional and psychological aspects of a child's problem. At this point, we must expand our armamentarium by bringing psychoeducational specialists into our clinical service and training programs. These persons, with a background in special education, should be integral members of our staffs, just as social workers and psychologists are. At our clinic we have found that the psychoeducational specialist has been invaluable in terms of the diagnostic assessment of a child's current learning skills and deficits, and in the development of a comprehensive therapeutic and remedial program. The specialist also sensitizes staff to the recognition of learning problems, arranges tutorial experiences, and serves in a school liaison role. The Day Diagnostic Center (see Chapter 6) is an even more sophisticated example of joint psychiatric/educational planning and intervention.

Bill: And now one final task for our child psychiatrist of the future. He is likely to have an administrative or managerial role, at the level of both the individual case or the development of a program. Throughout this book, we have commented on various programs, many of which have had major components of administration. A child psychiatrist has received little in his training up to this point to prepare him for administrative or managerial activities, how to develop a program, how to manage a clinic, how to deal with items such as budgets and personnel policies. This kind of subject matter, ultimately related to funding, has often been seen as too demeaning for professional discussion, yet the future of many programs is just as dependent, or more dependent, on business acumen than it is on goodwill or noble intentions. Even at the clinical level of the individual patient, certain managerial skills are important. When we talk especially about the severely disturbed and multiply handicapped child, we know that helping this child and his family will require a multitude of skills: pediatric, neurological, special educational, physiotherapeutic, and rehabilitational. And yet, we rarely learn how to analyze what is needed and how to help orchestrate the necessary programs for children and families who are in this situation. This is not to imply that we should be the main or only conductors of such an orchestra, but at least if we are to be involved in the role of helping, we ought to have had some experience in how to do it.

DAY TWO: A BACKWARD GLANCE

Marc: Yesterday we spoke of our beliefs regarding child psychiatry and offered several prescriptions for the future. In this, our final chapter, we can be more personal and more reflective. For most of the past decade, we have been engaged in the kind of programs we have described. Let's look back at them from our current vantage point. How do we feel about our work? What happened to these programs? Are the ideas behind them still valid? What impact did these programs have on us? How did we change, or have we? Let's take a look at these questions.

Bill: Okay. Looking back, even though most of our work was done separately, I think our experiences were similar in many ways. We were naïve and idealistic, two child psychiatrists just out of training, politically liberal, trying to change the world. No, I think that is too grandiose. We were trying to change a small segment of it. As we saw it, we were trying to change the system that we had contact with, and most of our contact was with the schools. We

were intruders on someone else's turf. We considerably underestimated and were ignorant of the problems we would encounter. I
think we were aware from the beginning that it was not just a
simple matter of generalizing from the clinical skills paradigm to
the institutional one, and we were aware that it is difficult to work
in an unfamiliar setting. We knew how to handle ourselves with
patients, both children and their families, in the mental health
clinic. We were receivers of somebody else's extrusion process,
and people came to us and we did our job inside four walls of our
structure, and then these people went out into the real world to ply
or use the effects of our treatment, hopefully. At least that is one
way of oversimplifying what we did. We certainly did not know
the rules of the game when we went outside of our previous territorial experience. I think we felt that our good will and, I suppose,
our knowledge of human psychology and behavior, albeit most of
it from a point of view of disturbance and deviance, would carry us
through. I do think we were aware, though, that we were learners,
that we were starting out as strangers, not only intruders but
strangers in another territory, and we were at times, at least in our
words if not in our actions, willing to learn about the other territory and the people who occupied it.

Marc: I remember that the school where I had my first school consultation experience was architectually very similar to the school
where I had spent my own elementary grade years. It had been
built at about the same time as my own school and was laid out in
a very similar plan. When I first went there, I felt like a fourth or
fifth grader who had to pass some kind of test with the principal
and teachers. I soon began to divide the school staff into
"goodies" and "baddies." The goodies said all the right things
about the relationship between education and mental health, the
needs of children, the effects of poverty, and the importance of
communication. The baddies spoke of discipline, grades,
suspension, and truancy, and they appeared to be the kinds of
people who often are simplistically labeled "racist."

Bill: Yes, I think one of the mistakes we made at that time was that we
were too much involved with the personality of the individual,
looking at him as a clinical phenomenon, rather than within the
whole social matrix in terms of roles that he had to play, given his
responsibility and office. And before we sound too penitent or
begin to flagellate ourselves with the 20-20 vision of hindsight, we
should acknowledge that we were also caught up in the times. The
spirit of the times had bred the "War on Poverty." The issue of

civil rights had moved into the streets and had evolved into a much more outspoken and polarizing kind of discussion that focused on black consciousness and white racism. There was a great deal of effort and considerable rhetoric aimed at changing the social system from many points of view. This included the political system, the military draft system, the class system, and certainly the educational system. We failed, however, to distinguish between the system as a symbol and the concrete aspects of the system. We were part of a legion of workers, do-gooders, and tub-thumpers, who were expected to be social engineers and pioneers of the new humanism. We were certainly fighting a relatively significant war within our own discipline with the traditionalists or "old fogies." So our excesses were probably no worse than most, nor was our naïvete. I agree with your distinction about goodies and baddies. It was an easy way to deal with people, and it helped foster a certain kind of internal cohesion among those who were trying to change an inflexible system, and it was certainly a superficial way of dealing with other people. I think in our clinical role, we would have been more appreciative of the complexities of the individual and his disturbance or the family and its problems. I want to make a comment later about how our social experience has, in turn, affected our clinical role. We are now talking about the reverse.

Marc: There was one particular principal, a "goodie" who said all the "right things," that is, the kinds of things we have talked about in this book. However, he *did* all the wrong things. He did not keep appointments, he pretended to give other people authority to make decisions, he allowed for very little initiative, and he did not follow through on anything. Perhaps as psychiatrists who are trained to value the spoken word so highly, we are too easily captivated by what people say rather than by what they do.

Bill: Well, I bet you each of our "favorite" principals has some favorite mental health consultants that he could talk about at considerable length. But I would like to get back to one of the questions raised at the beginning of our discussion today. How has our experience changed us?

Marc: My experience has made me appreciate the limits of my craft. For instance, there were aspects of my previous training in child psychiatry which were helpful to me—an understanding of communication, and an appreciation of my own reaction to situations—but I also learned that there was much I did not know, especially in terms of specific strategies and techniques to implement my ideas.

Bill: I think I learned, and I mean learned or really experienced in an
emotional sense, much more about the real lives of our patients. It
came through time after time, the difference between the office
experience and what we learned when we were in a school, talking
with DPW workers, making home visits, or sitting down with incentive specialists trying to figure out what was happening. In the
office we see only a small, and sometimes artificial, segment of the
reality of our patient's lives. And, in fact, that is what they are.
They are "patients" and we see the patient aspect of their lives and
focus on it. At least that is what I think our clinical training taught
us to do. Not only our clinical training in psychiatry but the whole
medical perspective of focusing on the sick part, whether it be a
"cardiac," a "diabetic," or a "neurotic" child. When we see
people at home, at school, or when we talk to their teachers about
them, we really begin to get a palpable sense of what the total life
of these children is like. We also get a fuller picture of the life of
the school itself. I know this may sound somewhat trite, and it
has been said before, but when you see children where they live
and act, you really get some sense of *their* life, in contrast to the
office where they fit into *our* life.

Marc: We also get a much better appreciation of what they are up
against. We know so little about what makes some children survive and do well in adversity and others fail. And along with that,
when you are out "there" and not in your office, you become fully
aware of the dilemmas of teachers, parents, and all those who deal
with children. For instance, how do you teach 35 pupils, many of
them at different achievement levels, in a rundown school. It is a
humbling experience to see that, and you certainly come away
feeling that you do not have any precious, neat answers, that you
can deliver from the protection and isolation of your office.

Bill: Let's talk more about what effect being out in the other man's turf
has had on us, rather than what effect we have had on the social
system. One of the things that I am impressed with is the change
in the way I think and talk about whatever it is that we try to help
with in terms of disturbance, emotional problems, and family
difficulties. I find that I am now using much more simple speech
and am much more descriptive in my clinical work, whether I am
describing it to myself, to another colleague or to a trainee. I find
that the jargon I once treasured and used is now no longer useful.
It seems to get in the way, and implies a degree of knowledge, or
perhaps a set of beliefs that I no longer hold nor find useful. I find
also that the experience out there has helped me get a little clearer

picture of what strengths and assets mean. I no longer see myself in the clinical sense as unraveling the complex mysteries of the psyche or mining the deep layers of the unconscious processes.

Marc: So rather than talk about how you are going to treat someone "for an Oedipal problem by analyzing his transference neurosis," you might say, "This child is having a hard time growing up and he needs some help." But just so we do not set up psychoanalysis as the straw man, another "baddie," I think we can put it in perspective by saying that there are certain principles and processes in analytic theory that have validity. However, it is a question of how much emphasis one gives them, how much time one puts into that kind of endeavor. For instance, I think I have seen instances in which the therapy *becomes* life, rather than the therapy being used to help someone in various aspects of his or her life.

But beyond that, beyond the influence that our experience out in the community has had on us as individual clinicians, I think we have fallen short in other areas. For example, we have written at some length about the organizational problems of various social institutions. I do not think, however, we have examined our own mental health clinics with the same degree of scrutiny. We have talked about them in a limited fashion in various chapters, but I know that we would be very resistant if any "intruder" came into *our* agencies and tried to get us to "do a better job," implicitly or explicitly, as we tried to do on someone else's grounds.

Bill: Perhaps, what we need are more people from alien fields, outsiders coming into different agencies with different perspectives. It reminds me of the fox in the chicken coop or the flea in the shirt (see glossary Table 1.1) that can have a beneficial as well as a pernicious influence, depending on how the fox or the flea happens to operate, or the response of the inhabitants of the coop or the shirt. At any rate, do you think that our approach is still valid?

Marc: Admitting its shortcomings, I still think it makes sense to deal as much as possible with those persons who are in caretaking positions vis-à-vis children and to try to influence in some small way the attitudes and beliefs of those persons and the institutions in which they function. This may no longer be a particularly practical viewpoint, in view of the funding cutbacks in the human service areas. And let's keep in mind that insufficient funds did cause the end of some of our programs, such as Parent Education and the consultation to the Department of Public Welfare. The Incentive Specialist program expired when the grant ran out, and some of the programs in which we tried new methods are still going on, such as the Black Brother Program and Mental Health Assistant Program. And other programs modeled on the ones we have described have been started. Even if there is less money available for particular programs in the future, the ultimate test of our efforts may be whether we can convey our attitudes and philosophy to our students.

Bill: I think that another major feature of our approach is still useful. We have emphasized a role development for mental health workers that puts a premium on skill building based on interest and talent rather than on professional background or training. I think this approach will continue to gain acceptance and application aided ironically by the marked decrease in federal training funds and the increased emphasis on service accountability.

DAY THREE: PRIORITIES

Marc: Yesterday, we talked about certain changes in ourselves, while at the same time we were discussing how our programs attempted to change certain attitudes and beliefs in a small segment of the social system, for instance, the school. Now, let's talk about priorities at the national level in terms of the mental health needs of children. I bring up this point because I find it gives me considerable trouble when I attempt to discuss it coherently. You and I could both run down a list of about 10 or 20 areas which require attention. This has been done quite comprehensively in the Joint Commission's report,[6] and we could rather repetitiously and boringly recite a litany of programs that are needed in terms of early intervention, nutrition, prenatal care, early detection, case finding, family income assistance, genetic counseling, programs for working mothers, day care, educational improvement programs, expansion of clinical services, drug rehabilitation centers, and family life education. Now each of us might have his own particular preference for one particular program or another, but when you come right down to it, how do we, as a profession, decide about priorities?

Bill: Well, you know, Marc, as psychiatrists we are always touting the idea of facing reality and being able to appraise reality and we are always promoting that for our patients. I think we ought to take that message to heart ourselves. It seems to me that there is a certain set of "givens" at the national scene, including the following.

First, our economy is moving from a product "hardware" type of economy toward a service "software" economy. Accompanying that, and already visible, is a whole shift in the preoccupation of citizens and politicians alike. The skills, techniques, and approaches that made the product economy run are going to be shifted to the service economy. More and more considerations of cost-benefit ratios, accountability, and fiscal management are going to be applied to service institutions, including mental health institutions. More consumers, individually and as a large developing movement, are demanding that service be better, that it be less costly, and that it be more efficiently delivered. They are asking for the kinds of things that they asked for when they wanted better and more efficient cars or better and more efficient TV sets. Whether these demands are realistic and whether they can be fulfilled is something else again. But the fact is those are the kinds of demands and concerns that are being voiced.

Now mental health is an enterprise and it is getting to be a big enterprise. It's part of an even larger health enterprise. It is going to start being treated like a business and being subject to some of the expectations and criteria to which business is subjected. Consequently, there is, and will be, more direct control from outside the mental health enterprise by government through legal and administrative measures. More and more the political and bureaucratic mentality, methods and approaches will be applied. One can bemoan it, one can bewail it, one can wish it were not so, but that seems to be the "given" we have to deal with. We said yesterday that clinical skills in analyzing and understanding the dynamics of an individual patient were not very useful and have little coinage when applied to dealing with administrative, fiscal, and political matters, that is, the items of power. And the people in power will determine the "givens" under which mental health operates and will continue to operate. They will be setting the rules, and they will be setting the priorities with or without our help or concurrence. Let me add, lest I be misunderstood, that this is not a plea for a return to rockrib McKinleyism. This is a statement of how I see things, not as how I wish they were.

Marc: So if we are pious and virtuous, it is not going to be enough. We
        are really faced with a means problem, finding out how to get
        something done, rather than an ends problem. As I said before, we
        know what is desirable and necessary for the needs of children.
        Now to get it done by preaching may be helpful, but only if we are
        very effective preachers, à la Billy Graham, or if we are the fa-
        vorite preachers of the President, again à la Billy Graham. But be-
        yond preachers ("advocate" is the more favorite current term) we
        also have to be poolroom hustlers. To stretch the point, and hope-
        fully add a little bit of humor to this treatise, we might suggest
        that the next president of the American Psychiatric Association be
        a cross between Oral Roberts and Minnesota Fats.

Bill: Marc, your comment about being the President's preachers main-
        tains our religious analogy and makes an important point. The in-
        dividual person can have some influence, I think, on fulfilling
        priorities in several ways. For instance, individual men of power
        may have had certain experiences that predispose them to favor
        one kind of program over another, to push mental retardation as
        the Kennedys did, or polio prevention as Roosevelt did. Or one
        may personally know an important political figure, and thus
        influence program priorities and funding. But these are fortuitous
        events. One has to be born in the right place, go to the right
        schools, meet or marry the right people, or treat the right people
        successfully. Short of that, I do not think the individual person is
        that influential. I think one does come around to the issue of orga-
        nizational effectiveness or group effectiveness. One can join the
        consumer movement or a committee for human rights, and work
        as a citizen-professional in promoting those ends that we all agree
        are good, through certain means that may or may not be effective.
        One can become a more active member of the American Psy-
        chiatric Association and become more politically minded both
        within the organization and as an advocate for the organization
        before government committees regarding legislative proposals or
        administrative regulations. Or, some of us who have identities and
        roles connected with the university can operate through that route
        in attempting to assure that appropriate consideration is given to
        such issues as training and research, if those are the priorities one
        believes are important, and since those are the priorities that
        universities and training institutions have traditionally pushed.
        The point is, I think, that organizations are generally self-serving
        in the sense that they serve the interests of their members. They

try to preserve the status quo by means of negativism or attempt to influence government and other outside forces and make some trade-offs. The aim is to retain ability to set some terms for what jobs they will do and how they will do them.

Marc: The problem is that we and some of our colleagues are quite ambivalent about this kind of activity. We see politicking, committee work, and organizational business, as boring, at best, and occasionally demeaning. Also, I think, we tend to be suspicious of organizations, we like to freelance, and would rather think of ourselves as pursuing more erudite endeavors (such as writing this book). For instance, who wants to sit on a joint university-state planning committee, responsible for designing a new facility for retarded children, and worry about issues such as civil service codes, budget slots, hiring and firing procedures, and laundry and janitorial services. The question that we at least internally ask frequently is "Did I get 9 years of training beyond college for this?" You see, when you begin medical school, you may think of yourself as a future Freud, Curie, or Ehrlich (or all those people Paul Muni played in the movies), but then you find yourself having to do work that is similar to what one probably does in an advertising agency, furniture business, or supermarket.

Bill: Well, one of the things I think you are saying, and it is part of the "givens" or realities, is that as one moves up within the profession and outside of the strictly therapeutic role, one moves toward being a manager. It is kind of a common final pathway for a number of careers, whose members often do not start out with management skills. and therefore, we become amateur managers and usually do not like it because we are not good at it. We are not pros, and we are playing with pros or against them. The facts then are such that if one wants to influence the political process or the administrators or regulatory agencies, they one has to make a career choice. One choice involves going up the bureaucratic ladder in a state agency or university department and, through persistence and a degree of luck and skill, becoming a pro at being an administrator or manager. Or another route is the political one; one can run for office or in some way become connected with the political and professional organizational process. If we decide not to do those kinds of things, or if we are not lucky enough to be a personal friend or confidant of men in power, then we end up wishing things were different and playing the fruitless game of "ain't it awful."

DAY FOUR: RACE AND SELF

Bill: This is the last day of our retreat, and on Monday, it will be back
          to work and sin. After having reviewed our dialogues over the past
          few days, I find that we have omitted one highly significant issue.
          Much of our work was done in the late sixties and during that time
          racism and black identity were predominant social themes. Al-
          though we may have touched on this question tangentially in con-
          nection with our program descriptions, we have really not dis-
          cussed it in any specific particularized manner. After all, we are
          two white, middle class, child psychiatrists and most of our work,
          though not all of it, involved programs that dealt with poor, black
          children and their families. We did have some problems, problems
          with our consultees, our clients, and ourselves. Let's talk about
          them.

Marc: It might be worthwhile, at least as a start, to describe some of the
          salient characteristics of those of us who were white, middle class
          psychiatrists who began to work in black and poor areas. I think it
          is important that we keep emphasizing that the issues of poverty
          and class are as important as the issue of race in our discussions.
          (As one example, housing conflicts are often a reflection of the
          "have nots" threatening the "haves" a little. But the surface issue
          is black-white.) Anyway, I think as white, middle-class pro-
          fessionals, we approached our task as "a new challenge." We saw
          ourselves as well intentioned, as liberal, as feeling a social obli-
          gation perhaps to attend to the "unfinished business of society" as
          our technical competence and skills permitted. We also did not do
          it with great sacrifice of position, prestige, or income. So it was
          not some martyrish or highly altruistic self-sacrifice in which we
          were involved. I think we believed, and at times rightly, and at
          times wrongly, that our good intentions, or basic "humanity," and
          the skills we had learned about understanding of human behavior
          would carry us through. We believed we were prepared to deal
          with whatever we faced not only in terms of patient care but as we
          became more aware of the fundamental human issues that did re-
          volve around race and class. Well, we were not exactly knights on
          white chargers, but we probably did turn into Don Quixote's. Do
          you think we were motivated by guilt?

Bill: If by guilt you mean that I did something that I feel bad about,
          and I have to make up for it by engaging in my professional
          activities with a certain group of people as a way of expiation, I do
          not think so. One can always claim that that is what was uncon-

sciously motivating me and that I did not know about it, but that is the kind of unassailable assertion which passes beyond the realm of reasonable discourse.

Marc: I think it is fair to say that occasionally I did feel uncomfortable, sometimes quite uncomfortable, in various situations with blacks. I rarely felt this discomfort in dealing with black children and their families in the context of the doctor-patient relationship. It may very well be because I was somewhat insulated by my role identity as a so-called expert whom the family was consulting for help. But there is also something direct, immediate, and personal about that kind of contact which lowered the barriers against racial differences. I was also operating on my own "turf," using the clinical skills that I have been trained in, and I found that these skills could be applied to a variety of families in different circumstances.

Black-white questions became more important when I moved out of my office and into the schools. We have already gone on at great length about problems involved in implementing a school program. When the question on my whiteness came up in a school program which involved a black principal, black teachers, or black pupils, it was generally an issue that was added on to a number of issues. I was then working on someone else's turf, trying to accomplish some kind of organizational change within the school. My white identity in several instances was a problem, but it was very much part of the smorgasbord of a host of other problems that had less to do with my whiteness, and more to do with my role as consultant. For instance, if I, as a white child psychiatrist, had restricted myself to seeing individual children within a school program, much in the same way I see them in my office, I think there would have been very little difficulty. It was when I was trying to design an overall program with a black principal that the question of my "relevance" as a white person was raised. If I had been trying to design a similar program with a white principal, he too, might have raised a number of questions about "relevance," but not about my being white.

Bill: Let's try to be specific about "racism." If by racism one means the inherent and fixed belief or assumption that I as a white person, and also as a representative of the white race as it were, am intrinsically superior morally, physically, or psychologically than another person of the black race, based upon my whiteness versus his blackness, then I do not think that notion was a significant part of my mental equipment or of many white people that I worked with. However, if one means that I naïvely assumed that whiteness was not a particularly important characteristic of how I saw myself, and also how other people reacted to me, then I suppose the charge "racism" applies. What became explicit for me as I worked with black clients, but also more particularly as I worked with black colleagues, and as I struggled, as you say, with consultation programs in black schools, was an awareness that some of my attitudes and some of the ways that people reacted to me were conditioned and related to the fact that I was white.

Marc: What you are saying is that you, like me, were raised white in a white world, with white standards and white "givens." But it was only after we began working with blacks that we became aware not only of their blackness but of our whiteness. There are differences among people, and when we really become cognizant of those differences, we become uncomfortable because we begin questioning whether all of the standard approaches that we have used before need to be reexamined. I think we become more sensitized to other people's feelings, we begin to look at kinds of words we use, and there is no doubt that we probably overreact and do too much laundering and oversanitizing so that we do not offend anyone because of his class or color. It may well be that *that,* too, is a form of racism, but I really do not think so.

Bill: You know, it is not what you say, it is how you say it. When black people called themselves and were called negroes, I did not really call myself or see myself as white. When black people or at least some black people started calling themselves black and calling their own and our attention to that characteristic very explicitly, then I had to attend to that. In addition, I had to attend and face the issue of whiteness. It did polarize, it did make explicit what was implicit and covered over by a different kind of term. Negro is an abstract label; black is a concrete color and that makes a different impact.

And it is also important to be as careful as we can about terminology. I think lumping everything under the term *racism* is just as bad as the kind of lumping we do diagnostically, when everything is called *sickness*. We have to be precise about distinguishing various aspects of racism, or lack of consciousness about race, and what it implies or does not imply, and how it influences attitudes and behavior.

I would agree with you that as black people faced their own blackness and began to deal with it, and as they faced me with my whiteness, I became more self-conscious, more aware of how I was saying things, and what I was saying. In that sense I think there is a developmental process that occurs when one does encounter new awareness about oneself. I suppose it is very similar to a kind of a therapeutic awareness and development. Therefore, the recent term that blacks are using is the new "white consciousness." I do not know what that means in detail, but perhaps it refers to this developmental process.

Marc: When one begins to feel like a "whitey" either defensively or because one has been accused of racism, I think there are several responses that can occur. If I think I am being personally attacked on the grounds that I am white and cannot deal with blacks, I can say "Who, me?" and trot out all of my liberal credentials and attempt to prove that my vote for McGovern means that I love blacks, Indians, and all poor and minority groups. Or I can become counter-accusatory and say that blacks just do not understand whites. Or, I can become very "sympathetic," and say that I understand the roots of the hostility and empathize with the black plight. Or I can become "black," that is, adopt a black dialect, use jive expressions, and give the Afro handshake, and in a variety of ways make myself look silly as a white person trying to be black. Along with these "in" mannerisms, I can espouse an exceedingly vitriolic antiwhite philosophy directed at my own heritage and against "establishment" white institutions. This attitude is akin to that of the religious convert or reformed alcoholic who attacks all aspects of his former self.

Bill: Your last comment reminds me of a true-to-life anecdote in which a white psychiatrist made the comment to a black social worker that he, the black social worker, was not black enough in his attitudes. If that is not the height of pecksniffian arrogance, I don't know what is.

You spoke primarily of the doctor-patient relationship, and I would agree with the points you made. When we move into the consultative relationship where we come as representatives of an institution, a mental health center or clinic, to a school or community group, another institution, and when that institution also is staffed by a fair number of black people in positions of responsibility or whose clients are primarily black, the issue of black-white becomes somewhat different. I came from Temple's mental health center into schools and was seen as a symbolic representative again. I was an outsider, I was white and professional, and I also was connected with a suspect institution. This institution was seen by community members as one that engaged in oppressive behavior toward blacks and poor people. There was reason for this view of the parent institution which in the fifties and early sixties had dislocated large numbers of residents and paid no more attention to relocation than governmental or other academic institutions did at that time. Its medical services, although no worse than many others, were seen as being impersonal, indifferent, and unresponsive. The mental health center had committed itself to the training of black paraprofessionals as the primary therapists, and had been attempting to provide more extensive, effective, and responsible services to people who lived in the North Philadelphia community. Our intentions, our beginning gestures, or our good will did not immediately change our reputation nor the attitude that people who lived in the community had toward us. So with the Incentive Specialist Program, I found myself in the situation in which I was suspect because of the institution I was connected with, because I was an outsider, and because I was white. When we came into a predominantly black school, all the usual problems of a consultant were compounded with being white. As such we were perceived as ready to label black kids crazy, or to tell black administrators what to do, thus maintaining in their eyes the same old oppressive and exploitative relationship.

Marc: In the Incentive Specialist Program you also brought with you the baggage of a research design. An attempt at research can provide further ammunition to the charge of exploitation, since once again here were white professionals "studying" black people. Most of the articles in the mental health literature about black families are by white men. Most of the research has been done by whites, and a natural response by some segments of the black community would be to say, "You don't know anything about black life. We, the black people, are the experts. We do not need your studies. If you really want to do something, why don't you study your white racist brethren? We will take care of ourselves." And although one can be very honest, sincere, and professional about a research design, the fact remains that during that time, during the "War on Poverty," working with and doing research on blacks was fashionable. It would have been logical for blacks to view this sudden interest on the part of the white professional community with a fair degree of suspicion.

Bill: I think that again, putting the issue of black awareness in the context of the sixties, it was the first of several kinds of uprisings by underdogs of society versus top dogs. Students were another group that rose up against their administrators and their masters and called into question how things were done. More recently, and with a great deal of momentum, women have raised some fundamental issues about male-female relationships and have pointed out the inequities and injustices, social, personal, and psychological that they see have been put on them by a male-dominated society. So, in that context, the black rebellion was the first and one of the most important. It had generated a great deal of staying power in terms of calling into question the nature of the relationships between black and white, both at an individual and societal level. I think blacks and the other groups are calling into question the basic social contract. They want to have a part in making the terms for a new kind of contract rather than accepting the old terms as a God-given or permanently established way to do business together. Once this awareness developed in black people, their spokesmen said the unspeakable and began talking in plain language about such things as oppression and racism. Such talk gave encouragement to a large number of black people to express what they may not even have been able to clearly formulate before, or if formulated, they did not feel could be said. Thus, as a white person I did not realize the degree of suspicion and distrust that many black people have for white people, including myself, despite the cordiality, depth of affection, and friendship that some of these relationships have engendered.

Marc: And I think on the other side that I have tended to view individual blacks at times as symbols of the black race. Occasionally, at the very personal level, the symbolic differences disappear, but there are also times when they occur, somewhat surprisingly, or somewhat unexpectedly. This question of trying to separate the individual person from his symbolic representation brings us to another vital question. We are all guilty of the tendency to generalize. I know that is a trite statement, and it has been said before, but I think it is important to say it again. We are talking about the two of us and our experiences, and the experiences of some black principals, teachers, colleagues, and patients with us. We may think what we are saying is valid, but in the larger scheme of things, our experience is narrow, and I think we should caution against the blinders of reductionism.

Bill: If we take the notions that we have been discussing, that is, symbolism and generalization, we come on the topic of rhetoric and its influence in this phenomena of white-black relations. Rhetoric has numerous dictionary meanings, but I think that the ones that are most applicable here are those that relate to persuasive speech, verbosity, and bombast. It is probably the nature of rhetoric, at least as it has been used in the black experience and certainly in the antiwar movement and other experiences, to engage in the kind of reductionism that you spoke about. Issues are polarized. Persons and groups are seen as being either on one side or on the other. Assertions serve as evidence and polemic replaces reason. In such a climate, the opportunity for critical evaluation of positions is almost impossible. Criticism is taken by one side or the other as being a sign of one's intrinsic obstinancy, ignorance, or bad intent.

Marc: It is important to acknowledge the use of rhetoric for the primary consumers, that is, blacks speaking to blacks, making them aware of their history, and what has been done to them as a people and as individuals, and how it has been done and who has done it. What I find troublesome is when that same rhetoric becomes the only or primary approach between blacks and whites. When a white person says to a black person, "What do you mean by racism?" and is greeted with the response that the very fact that you asked that question is a symptom of racist mentality or ignorance, it seems to me that is where rhetoric is misused and not useful.

Similarly, when a white person in response to questions states that he views Malcolm X or Stokely Carmichael as merely demagogues, who are promoting self-aggrandizement by the use of racial feelings, this in turn partakes of the same sort of rhetoric or counter-rhetoric that maintains polarization and stifles discussion. Rhetoric is often used as a substitute for name calling and becomes a way of once again dividing people into "goodies" and "baddies." For instance, I may agree with another person's point of view, but it does not mean that I have to be a convert to all details of his ideology. And while we argue about whether or not I am a true believer, questions of strategies and tactics which might lead to the implementation of our shared views are obscured.

I think we have gone about as far with this discussion as we can. And what applies to our experience then as far as the black-white question is concerned may not be as applicable now. We have reviewed our own thoughts on this matter at some length and we are not really proposing any solution. In other parts of this book, we have talked about problems, but we have also talked about remedies. Those problems, however, had to do basically with questions of technique. The racial problem, however, is not a technical one, but rather a social, human, and personal problem.

Bill: I have just received a telephone message that we are both needed back at the clinic. You have an emergency budget meeting that has just been scheduled because one of the grants fell through, and I have to see a child suspended from school.

Marc: You mean we just can't sit here and be philosophers?

Bill: No, but maybe we can meet for lunch at the clinic tomorrow.

Marc: All right, see you at work.

REFERENCES

1. The Gospel according to St. Matthew 19:24
2. Hughes E: Good people and dirty work. Soc Probl 10:3–11, 1962
3. Stevenson G, Smith G: Child Guidance Clinics: A Quarter Century of Development. New York, The Commonwealth Fund, 1934
4. Witmer H : Psychiatric Clinics for Children. New York, The Commonwealth Fund, 1940, p 365
5. Hetznecker W, Forman MA: Community child psychiatry: evolution and development. Am J Orthopsychiatry 4:350–370, 1971
6. Report of the Joint Commission on Mental Health of Children. Crisis in child mental health: challenge for the 1970's. New York, Harper & Row, 1969

Index